Te of Dental Radiology

Textbook
of
Dental Radiology

Second Edition

Pramod John R BSc, BDS, MDS
Professor and Head
Department of Oral Medicine, Oral Diagnosis and Radiology
Amrita School of Dentistry
Amrita Institute of Medical Sciences and Research (A Constituent
Institution of Amrita Vishwa Vidyapeetham–A Deemed University)
Kochi, Kerala, India
Formerly, Associate Professor, Department of Oral Medicine and
Radiology, College of Dental Surgery, Kasturba Medical College,
Manipal and Mangalore and Professor and Head, Department of Oral
Medicine and Radiology, Mahatma Gandhi Government Dental
College and Hospital, Indira Nagar Complex, Puducherry, India

JAYPEE BROTHERS MEDICAL PUBLISHERS (P) LTD

Kochi • St. Louis (USA) • Panama City (Panama) • London (UK) • New Delhi
Ahmedabad • Bengaluru • Chennai • Hyderabad • Kolkata • Lucknow • Mumbai • Nagpur

Published by

Jitendar P Vij

Jaypee Brothers Medical Publishers (P) Ltd

Corporate Office

4838/24 Ansari Road, Daryaganj, **New Delhi** - 110002, India, Phone: +91-11-43574357
Fax: +91-11-43574314

Registered Office

B-3 EMCA House, 23/23B Ansari Road, Daryaganj, **New Delhi** - 110 002, India
Phones: +91-11-23272143, +91-11-23272703, +91-11-23282021, +91-11-23245672
Rel: +91-11-32558559, Fax: +91-11-23276490, +91-11-23245683
e-mail: jaypee@jaypeebrothers.com, Website: www.jaypeebrothers.com

Offices in India

- **Ahmedabad**, Phone: Rel: +91-79-32988717, e-mail: ahmedabad@jaypeebrothers.com
- **Bengaluru**, Phone: Rel: +91-80-32714073, e-mail: bangalore@jaypeebrothers.com
- **Chennai**, Phone: Rel: +91-44-32972089, e-mail: chennai@jaypeebrothers.com
- **Hyderabad**, Phone: Rel:+91-40-32940929, e-mail: hyderabad@jaypeebrothers.com
- **Kochi**, Phone: +91-484-2395740, e-mail: kochi@jaypeebrothers.com
- **Kolkata**, Phone: +91-33-22276415, e-mail: kolkata@jaypeebrothers.com
- **Lucknow**, Phone: +91-522-3040554, e-mail: lucknow@jaypeebrothers.com
- **Mumbai**, Phone: Rel: +91-22-32926896, e-mail: mumbai@jaypeebrothers.com
- **Nagpur**, Phone: Rel: +91-712-3245220, e-mail: nagpur@jaypeebrothers.com

Overseas Offices

- **North America Office, USA,** Ph: 001-636-6279734
  e-mail: jaypee@jaypeebrothers.com, anjulav@jaypeebrothers.com
- **Central America Office, Panama City, Panama,** Ph: 001-507-317-0160
  e-mail: cservice@jphmedical.com, Website: www.jphmedical.com
- **Europe Office, UK,** Ph: +44 (0) 2031708910, e-mail: info@jpmedpub.com

Textbook of Dental Radiology

© 2011, Pramod John R

This book has been published in good faith that the material provided by author is original. Every effort is made to ensure accuracy of material, but the publisher, printer and author will not be held responsible for any inadvertent error (s). In case of any dispute, all legal matters are to be settled under Delhi jurisdiction only.

First Edition: 1999
  Reprint: 2007
  Reprint: 2008

Second Edition: **2011**

ISBN 978-93-5025-079-2

Typeset at JPBMP typesetting unit
Printed at Rajkamal Electric Press, Plot No. 2, Phase-IV, Kundli, Haryana.

Dedicated

To
My Parents for their
Joy in my successes,
Compassion in my fallibility,
Encouragement in my academic pursuits,
Understanding in my mistakes,
Support when my steps falter,
And above all for making me what I am.

To
My Teachers for
Teaching me the values and virtues of life,
Opening new vistas of ever-broadening knowledge,
Taking me out of my ignorance,
Patience in teaching to make me understand,
Unselfishness in imparting knowledge,
And above all for helping me reach where I am.

In Memoriam

To
The Memory of my mother,
Smt Mercy
Who Left For Her Heavenly Abode
On 22nd November 2007

Preface to the Second Edition

I had written the first edition of the book, titled, *'Essentials of Dental Radiology'* at a time when foreign textbooks were flooding the market and the students were finding it hard to browse through the enormous volumes of these books during their preparation phase for the examination. The time constraint and the cost factor were unfavorable for the average student to buy all these books.

I was greatly encouraged by the warm reception the book received which stimulated me to do the revision of the book. I have added many photographs and the entire text material has been edited and rewritten to suit the requirement of the readers.

I have also taken the valuable inputs from and suggestions received from the readers and publishers. It is my confidence that the new visual appeal, presentation and format of the book would be liked by the readers. Suggestions for the improvement of the book and criticisms are whole-heartedly solicited.

Pramod John R

Preface to the First Edition

I have derived immense enthusiasm to write this book, titled, *'Essentials of Dental Radiology'* from the encouragement I received from the readers after the publication of my maiden effort, *'Handbook of Oral Medicine'*, published by Jaypee Brothers Medical Publishers Pvt. Ltd., New Delhi in 1998. The objectives of writing this book remain the same as that of my first book.

All the chapters in this book are written in conformity with the syllabi of various Indian universities. As yet there is no book available which satisfies the requirements of the various syllabi. In this context, I am sure that this book will be quite useful for any student of dentistry. I have tried to provide the essential material in all the chapters so that the undergraduate and postgraduate students will acquire adequate subject knowledge to face the examination. In the preparation of the contents, I have excluded certain unnecessary details. Additional information in these areas, especially to the postgraduate students, may be obtained from appropriate reference books that are freely available in the country.

I request the readers to point out any inadvertent errors or omissions and offer constructive criticism, if any, in modifying or improving the contents. Your opinion about this book is also solicited.

Pramod John R

Acknowledgments

My parents were a wonderful source of encouragement, without which I would not have reached where I am now. They stood by me at times of joy as well as grief. During the course of preparation of the second edition of this book, I lost my mother so untimely and unexpectedly. I am sure she is in her heavenly abode and looking down on me. My daughter Priya deserves a special acknowledgment for all the joy and happiness she spreads at home.

I am greatly indebted to my *alma mater*, the College of Dental Surgery (a constituent college of Manipal Academy of Higher Education, Manipal—a Deemed University), where I was a student and served as a faculty for a lengthy period of time. The teachers I had there instilled in me the quest to learn more and more and also to pursue the less preferred path of academics as a career. I greatly remember the wonderful teachers I had there and to name a few, Dr MK Manjunath, Dr MR Vijay Raghavan, Dr Shobha Tandon, Dr Dileep R Gadevar, Dr GS Kumar and Dr Mahalinga Bhat.

I greatly appreciate and express my special thanks to my sister Dr Jayasree VM for helping me in correcting the proof and also for standing behind me as a source of strength and encouragement.

"Knowledge is of two kinds: we know a subject ourselves or we know where we can find information upon it", so wrote Boswell in 'Life of Samuel Johnson'. I greatly acknowledge the authors of various books that I have used as reference material. Their willingness to share the knowledge is greatly appreciated.

I am especially thankful to Shri Jitendar P Vij of Jaypee Brothers Medical Publishers (P) Ltd., New Delhi, India for all the encouragement as well as for bringing out this book in an excellent form.

I would like to thank all those who were involved directly or indirectly in the task of bringing out this book.

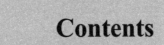

Contents

Chapter 1

History of Radiation

- *Introduction*
- *Discovery of X-radiation*
- *Chronology of Events in the Evolution of Dental Radiology*

Nothing in education is so astonishing as the amount of ignorance it accumulates in the form of inert facts.

– Henry B Adams

INTRODUCTION

The application of x-rays plays a vital role in the practice of dentistry as radiographs are required for a majority of the patients either as part of routine examination, diagnostic purpose, treatment planning or for follow-up evaluation of the patients. Radiographs are important in the routine investigation of dental caries and its sequelae, evaluation of periodontal diseases, identification of osseous pathologies such as cysts and tumors as well as in the evaluation of traumatic injuries involving the jaws and facial bones. Radiographs are also useful in the evaluation of growth and development. From the foregoing it is very clear that radiographs are sometimes referred to as the main diagnostic aids of the clinician.

Passing the x-rays through a structure to be examined and capturing the resultant image on a photographic emulsion of the film make a radiographic image. The number of x-rays reaching the film determines the overall exposure or blackening of the emulsion. Hard and mineralized structures absorb a great deal of radiation, whereas the soft tissues permit the passage of x-rays. The image thus produced is called as latent image as the film has to be chemically processed for converting the latent or invisible image into a permanent and visible image. The image that is produced by radiography is a two-dimensional image of the three-dimensional structure radiographed.

The amount of radiation absorbed (attenuated) by the structures determines the radiodensity of the shadows.

- The white or radiopaque areas represent dense structures
- The black or radiolucent areas represent structures that permitted the passage of x-rays to cast an image
- Gray shadows represent structures that have variably absorbed the x-rays.

Though the image quality is under the influence of various parameters acting alone or in combination, the various factors having an influence on the image formation can be summarized as follows:

- Number of x-ray photons passing through the structure
- The energy or intensity of the x-ray photons
- The exposure time or the period during which the x-rays were produced
- The size and shape of the object
- The thickness or density of the object
- The position of the object and film
- The sensitivity of the x-ray film.

KEY DEFINITIONS

Radiation

Radiation is a form of energy, carried by waves or stream of particles.

X-radiation

X-radiation is a high-energy radiation produced by the collision of a beam of electrons with a metal target in an x-ray tube.

X-ray

X-ray is a beam of energy that has the power to penetrate substances and record the resultant image on a photographic film.

Radiology

Radiology is the medical science that deals with the study of radiation and its use, radioactive substances and other forms of radiant energy in the diagnosis and treatment of diseases.

Radiograph

Radiograph is an image on a film, which is visible when viewed under transillumination, produced by the passage of x-rays through an object or body.

Radiography

Radiography is the art and science of making radiographs by the exposure of photographic films to x-rays.

Dental Radiology

Dental radiology is that area of dentistry, which is concerned with the study of radiation and its use; for the evaluation of teeth, their associated structures and facial and cranial bones.

Dental Radiograph

Dental radiograph is an image on a film showing the teeth and associated structures when viewed under transillumination.

DISCOVERY OF X-RADIATION

Wilhelm Conrad Roentgen (pronounced as 'ren-ken'), a Bavarian Physicist on November 8, 1895 discovered x-rays. Roentgen named these rays as x-rays due to the unknown nature and properties of these rays at the time of their discovery. The symbol 'x' is used in mathematics to represent an unknown quantity. X-rays are a form of high-energy electromagnetic radiation and are part of the electromagnetic spectrum.

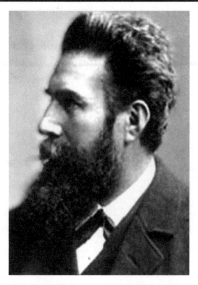

Fig. 1-1: Wilhelm Conrad Roentgen

Wilhelm Conrad Roentgen—Brief Biography (Fig. 1-1)

Wilhelm Conrad Roentgen was born on March 27, 1845, at Lennep in the Lower Rhine Province of Germany, as the only child of a merchant and manufacturer of cloth. His mother was Charlotte Constanze Frowein of Amsterdam, a member of an old Lennep family, which had settled in Amsterdam.

When he was three years old, his family moved to Apeldoorn in The Netherlands, where he went to the Institute of Martinus Herman van Doorn, a boarding school. He did not show any special aptitude, but showed a love of nature and was fond of roaming in the open country and forests. He was especially apt at making mechanical contrivances, a characteristic which remained with him also in later life. In 1862, he entered a technical school at Utrecht, where he was however unfairly expelled, accused of having produced a caricature of one of the teachers, which was in fact done by someone else.

He then entered the University of Utrecht in 1865 to study physics. Not having attained the credentials required for a regular student, and hearing that he could enter the Polytechnic at Zurich by passing its examination, he passed this and began studies there as a student of mechanical engineering. He attended the lectures given by Clausius and also worked in the laboratory of Kundt. Both Kundt and Clausius exerted great influence on his development. In 1869 he received PhD from the University of Zurich, was appointed assistant to Kundt and went with him to Würzburg in the same year, and three years later to Strasbourg.

In 1874, he qualified as Lecturer at Strasbourg University and in 1875, he was appointed Professor in the Academy of Agriculture at Hohenheim in Wurtemberg. In 1876 he returned to Strasbourg as Professor of Physics, but three years later he accepted the invitation to the Chair of Physics in the University of Giessen.

After having declined invitations to similar positions in the Universities of Jena (1886) and Utrecht (1888), he accepted it from the University of Würzburg (1888), where he succeeded Kohlrauschund found among his colleagues Helmholtz and Lorenz. In 1899 he declined an offer to the Chair of Physics in the University of Leipzig, but in 1900, he accepted it in the University of Munich, by special request of the Bavarian government, as successor of E Lommel. Here he remained for the rest of his life, although he was offered, but declined, the Presidency of the Physikalisch-Technische Reichsanstalt at Berlin and the Chair of Physics of the Berlin Academy.

Roentgen's first work was published in 1870, dealing with the specific heats of gases, followed a few years later by a paper on the thermal conductivity of crystals. Among other problems he studied were the electrical and other characteristics of quartz; the influence of pressure on the refractive indices of various fluids; the modification of the planes of polarized light by electromagnetic influences; the variations in the functions of the temperature and the compressibility of water and other fluids; the phenomena accompanying the spreading of oil drops on water.

Roentgen's name, however, is chiefly associated with his discovery of the rays that he called x-rays. In 1895 he was studying the phenomena accompanying the passage of an electric current through a gas of extremely low pressure. Previous work in this field had already been carried out by J Plucker (1801-1868), JW Hittorf (1824-1914), CF Varley (1828-1883), E Goldstein (1850-1931), Sir William Crookes (1832-1919), H Hertz (1857-1894) and Ph Von Lenard (1862-1947), and by the work of these scientists the properties of cathode rays, the name given by Goldstein to the electric current established in highly rarefied gases by the very high tension electricity generated by Ruhmkorff's induction coil, had become well-known. Roentgen's work on cathode rays led him, however, to the discovery of a new and different kind of rays.

On the evening of November 8, 1895, he found that, if the discharge tube is enclosed in a sealed, thick black carton to exclude all light, and if he worked in a dark room, a paper plate covered on one side with barium platinocyanide placed in the path of the rays became fluorescent even when it was as far as two meters from the discharge tube. During subsequent experiments he found that objects of different thicknesses interposed in the path of the rays showed variable transparency to them when recorded on a photographic plate. When he immobilized for some moments the hand of his wife in the path of the rays over a photographic plate, he observed after development of the plate an image of his wife's hand which showed the shadows thrown by the bones of her hand and that of a ring she was wearing, surrounded by the penumbra of the flesh, which was more permeable to the rays and therefore threw a fainter shadow. This was the first "roentgenograms" ever taken. In further experiments, Roentgen showed that the new rays are produced by the impact of cathode rays on a material object. Because their nature was then unknown, he gave them the name x-rays. Later, Max von Laue and his pupils showed that they are of the same electromagnetic nature as light, but differ from it only in the higher frequency of their vibration.

Numerous honors were showered upon him. In several cities, streets were named after him, and a complete list of prizes, medals, honorary doctorates, honorary and corresponding memberships of learned societies in Germany as well as abroad, and other honors would fill a whole page of this book. In spite of all this, Roentgen retained the characteristic of a strikingly modest and reticent man. Throughout his life he retained his love of nature and outdoor occupations. Many vacations were spent at his summer home at Weilheim, at the foot of the Bavarian Alps, where he entertained his friends and went on many expeditions into the mountains. He was a great mountaineer and more than once got into dangerous situations. Amiable and courteous by nature, he always understood the views and difficulties of others. He was always shy of having an assistant, and preferred to work alone. He built much of the apparatus he used with great ingenuity and experimental skill.

Roentgen married Anna Bertha Ludwig of Zurich, whom he had met in the café run by her father. She was a niece of the poet Otto Ludwig. They got married in 1872 in Apeldoorn, The Netherlands. They had no children, but in 1887 adopted Josephine Bertha Ludwig, then aged 6, daughter of Mrs. Roentgen's only brother. Four years after his wife's death, Roentgen died at Munich on February 10, 1923, due to carcinoma of the intestine.

History of Radiography

X-rays were discovered in 1895, by Wilhelm Conrad Roentgen (1845-1923, see the biographical sketch) who was a Professor at Wurzburg University in Germany. Like most of the scientific discoveries, even the discovery of x-rays was accidental at a time when Roentgen was experimenting with the production of cathode rays. Cathode rays are nothing but stream of electrons. For his experiment, he used the following:

- Vacuum tube
- An electrical current
- Special screens covered with a material, which fluoresces when exposed to radiation.

While experimenting in his darkened laboratory with a cathode ray tube, Roentgen noticed a faint and fluorescent glow coming from a table kept several feet away on which the fluorescent screens were kept. It was readily apparent to him that the cathode rays could never travel that far. This curious scientific observation prompted him to conclude that these rays were different and hence he named these rays as 'x-rays'. The tube that Roentgen was working with consisted of a glass envelope (bulb) with positive and negative electrodes encapsulated in it. The air in the tube was evacuated, and when a high voltage was applied, the tube produced a fluorescent glow. Roentgen shielded the tube with heavy black paper, and discovered a green-colored fluorescent light generated by a material located a few feet away from the tube.

He concluded that a new type of rays was being emitted from the tube. This ray was capable of passing through the heavy paper covering and exciting the phosphorescent materials in the room. He found that the new ray could pass through most substances casting shadows of solid objects. Roentgen also discovered that the ray could pass through the tissue of humans, but not bones and metal objects. One of Roentgen's first experiments late in 1895 was a film of the hand of his wife, Bertha (Fig. 1-2). It is interesting that the first use of x-rays were for an industrial (not medical) application, as Roentgen produced a radiograph of a set of weights in a box to show his colleagues.

Roentgen's discovery was a scientific bombshell, and was received with extraordinary interest by both scientists and laymen. Scientists everywhere could duplicate his experiment because the cathode tube was very well known during this

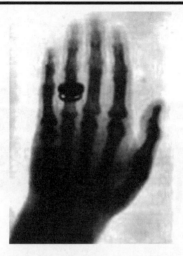

Fig. 1-2: The radiograph taken by Roentgen
of his wife Bertha Roentgen's hand

period. Many scientists dropped other lines of research to pursue the mysterious rays. Newspapers and magazines of the day provided the public with numerous stories, some true, others fanciful, about the properties of the newly discovered rays.

Public fancy was caught by this invisible ray that had the ability to pass through solid matter, and, in conjunction with a photographic plate, provided a picture of the bones and internal body parts. Scientific curiosity arose by the demonstration of wavelength of x-rays which is shorter than light. This generated new possibilities in physics, and for investigating the structure of matter. Much enthusiasm was generated about potential applications of x-rays as an aid in medicine and surgery. Within a month after the announcement of the discovery, several medical radiographs had been made in Europe and in the United States, which were used by surgeons to guide them in their work. In June 1896, only 6 months after Roentgen announced his discovery, x-rays were being used by battlefield physicians to locate bullets in wounded soldiers.

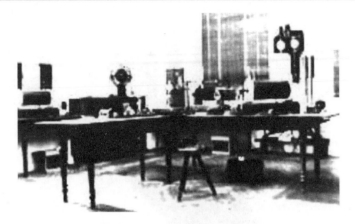

Fig. 1-3: Roentgen's laboratory

Prior to 1912, x-rays were used little outside the realms of medicine and dentistry, though some x-ray pictures of metals were produced. The reason that x-rays were not used in industrial application before this date was because the x-ray tubes (the source of the x-rays) broke down under the voltages required to produce rays of satisfactory penetrating power for industrial purposes. However, that changed in 1913 when the high vacuum x-ray tubes designed by Coolidge became available. The high vacuum tubes were an intense and reliable x-ray source, operating at energies up to 100,000 volts.

In 1922, industrial radiography took another step forward with the advent of the 200,000-volt x-ray tube that allowed radiographs of thick steel parts to be produced in a reasonable amount of time. In 1931, General Electric Company developed 1,000,000 volt x-ray generators, providing an effective tool for industrial radiography. That same year, the American Society of Mechanical Engineers (ASME) permitted x-ray approval of fusion welded pressure vessels that further opened the door to industrial acceptance and use (Fig. 1-3).

A Second Source of Radiation

Shortly after the discovery of x-rays, another form of penetrating rays was discovered. In 1896, French scientist Henri Becquerel discovered natural radioactivity. Many scientists of that period were working with cathode rays, and other scientists were gathering evidence on the theory that the atom could be subdivided. Some of the researches showed that certain types of atoms disintegrate by themselves. It was Henri Becquerel who discovered this phenomenon while investigating the properties of fluorescent minerals. Becquerel was researching the principles of fluorescence, wherein certain minerals glow (fluoresce) when exposed to sunlight. He utilized photographic plates to record this fluorescence.

One of the minerals Becquerel worked with was a uranium compound. On a day when it was too cloudy to expose his samples to direct sunlight, Becquerel stored some of the compound in a drawer with his photographic plates. Later when he developed these plates, he discovered that they were fogged (exhibited exposure to light). Becquerel wondered as to what would have caused this fogging. He knew he had wrapped the plates tightly before using them, so the fogging was not due to stray light. In addition, he noticed that only the plates that were in the drawer with the uranium compound were fogged. Becquerel concluded that the uranium compound gave off a type of radiation that could penetrate heavy paper and expose photographic film. Becquerel continued to test samples of uranium compounds and determined that the source of radiation was the element uranium. Becquerel's discovery was, unlike that of the x-rays, virtually unnoticed by laymen and scientists alike. Relatively few scientists were interested in Becquerel's findings. It was not until the discovery of radium by the Curies two years later that interest in radioactivity became widespread.

While working in France at the time of Becquerel's discovery, Polish scientist Marie Curie became very interested in his work. She suspected that a uranium ore known as pitchblende contained other radioactive elements. Marie and her husband, French scientist Pierre Curie, started looking for these other elements. In 1898, the Curies discovered another radioactive element in pitchblende, and named it 'polonium' in honor of Marie Curie's native homeland. Later that year, the Curie discovered another radioactive element which they named radium, or "shining element". Both polonium and radium were more radioactive than uranium. Since these discoveries, many other radioactive elements have been discovered or produced.

Radium became the initial industrial gamma ray source. The material allowed castings up to 10 to 12 inches thick to be radiographed. During World War II, industrial radiography grew tremendously as part of the Navy's shipbuilding program. In 1946, man-made gamma ray sources such as cobalt and iridium became available. These new sources were far stronger than radium and were much less expensive. The man-made sources rapidly replaced radium, and use of gamma rays grew quickly in industrial radiography.

Health Concerns

The science of radiation protection, or "health physics" as it is more properly called, grew out of the parallel discoveries of x-rays and radioactivity in the closing years of the 19th century. Experimenters, physicians, laymen, and physicists alike set-up x-ray generating apparatuses and proceeded about their labors with a lack of concern regarding potential dangers. Such a lack of concern is quite understandable, for there was nothing in previous experience to suggest that x-rays would in any way be hazardous. Indeed, the opposite was the case, for who would suspect that a ray similar to light but unseen, unfelt, or otherwise undetectable by the senses would be damaging to a person? More likely, or so it seemed to some, x-rays could be beneficial for the body.

Inevitably, the widespread and unrestrained use of x-rays led to serious injuries. Often injuries were not attributed to x-ray exposure, in part because of the slow onset of symptoms, and because there was simply no reason to suspect x-rays as the cause. Some early experimenters did tie x-ray exposure and skin burns together. The first warning of possible adverse effects of x-rays came from Thomas Edison, William J Morton, and Nikola Tesla who each reported eye irritations from experimentation with x-rays and fluorescent substances.

Today, it can be said that radiation ranks among the most thoroughly investigated causes of disease. Although much still remains to be learned, more is known about the mechanisms of radiation damage on the molecular, cellular, and organ system than is known for most other health stressing agents. Indeed, it is precisely this vast accumulation of quantitative dose-response data that enables health physicists to specify radiation levels so that medical, scientific, and industrial uses of radiation may continue at levels of risk no greater than, and frequently less than, the levels of risk associated with any other technology.

X-rays and gamma rays are electromagnetic radiation of exactly the same nature as light, but of much shorter wavelength. Wavelength of visible light is on the order of 6000 angstroms while the wavelength of x-rays is in the range of one angstrom and that of gamma rays is 0.0001 angstrom. This very short wavelength is what gives x-rays and gamma rays their power to penetrate materials that light cannot. These electromagnetic waves are of a high energy level and can break chemical bonds in materials they penetrate. If the irradiated matter is living tissue, the breaking of chemical bonds may result in altered structure or a change in the function of cells. Early exposures to radiation resulted in the loss of limbs and even lives. Men and women researchers collected and documented information on the interaction of radiation and the human body. This early information helped science understand how electromagnetic radiation interacts with living tissue. Unfortunately, much of this information was collected at great personal expense.

CHRONOLOGY OF EVENTS IN THE EVOLUTION OF DENTAL RADIOLOGY

Contributions of many scientists had paved the way for the evolution of dental radiology as a diagnostic science. Considerable improvizations of the previously crude equipments have also taken place. The earlier equipments were using a higher exposure time for getting the image. However, the knowledge about the harmful effects of x-radiation has helped in the designing of equipments which required less exposure time. It must also be emphasized that quite a lot of research activities are going on in the development of newer imaging modalities that could truly revolutionize the science of dental radiology. The chronology of these events in the evolution of dental radiology is summarized and given below.

1770s   William Morgan and Jean A Nolet experimented on electric (spark) discharges in partially evacuated glass vessels.

1821   Michael Faraday conducted studies on electric discharges and fluorescence of the gas present in an evacuated glass tube. This was then considered to be a fourth state of matter, other than the solid, liquid, and gaseous states.

1831   Michael Faraday described electromagnetic induction.

1861   William Crookes described that the cathode rays have momentum and energy and these rays were identified to be charged particles.

1861   Lenard proposed inverse square law pertaining to the cathode rays.

1880s   Description of Edison effect (emission of electrons from a hot filament) by Thomas Alva Edison.

1895   On November 8, 1895 Wilhelm Conrad Roentgen discovered x-rays.

1895   Jean Perrin proposed that cathode rays are negatively charged particles.

1896   John Joseph Thompson measured the velocity of cathode rays and the ratio between their charge and mass.

1896   William TG Morton, a dentist, announced that it is possible to take radiographs of the teeth.

1896   Dr Edmund C Kells discovered his own x-ray apparatus and described a technique for radiographing the teeth and the jaws. He also proposed the principle of keeping the film and object at right angles to the source of x-ray.

1896   Frank Harrison, an English dentist made dental radiographs with 10 minutes of exposure time. His images could differentiate the tooth structure and pulp chamber. He also reported the harmful effects of radiation.

1896   Wilhelm Koenig in Frankfurt made 14 dental radiographs.

1896   Dr Otto Walkoff made radiographs of the molars with an exposure time of 25 minutes.

1896   William J Morton used roll film.

1901   Roentgen was awarded the Nobel Prize in Physics.

1903   Kells described time-temperature method of film processing.

1904   Weston A Price, a Cleveland dentist, described paralleling technique and bisecting-angle technique.

1910   Franklin W McCormack proposed long distance technique.

1913   William D Coolidge, an electrical engineer, developed first hot cathode x-ray tube with tungsten filament.

1913   Dental x-ray packets consisted of glass photographic plates or films cut into small pieces and hand-wrapped.

1913   Wrapped and moisture-proof dental film packet containing two films were introduced in the market.

1917   Howard Riley Raper introduced angle meter.

1918   Coolidge made a tube with leaded glass tube, which served as a radiation shield.

1918   Eastman Kodak Company developed a darkroom with processing tanks.

1918   Rollins described collimation, intensifying screens, and the necessity of draping the patient with protective aprons for radiographic examination.

1919   Films were packed by machines.

1920	First machine-made periapical film was available in the market.
1920	Franklin W McCormack used the paralleling technique in dental radiography.
1923	A miniature version of the x-ray tube was placed inside the head of an x-ray machine by Victor X-Ray Corporation of Chicago.
1924	Films were produced with the emulsion coated on both the sides.
1924	Inflammable cellulose nitrate was replaced by non-inflammable cellulose triacetate.
1925	Raper proposed bitewing technique for the detection of interproximal caries.
1933	A new dental x-ray machine with improved features was manufactured by General Electric Company.
1937	Donald McCormack proposed long distance paralleling technique.
1947	Long cone paralleling technique was proposed by F Gordon Fitzgerald.
1949	American Academy of Dental Radiology was formed.
1957	Variable kilo voltage machine was introduced.
1960s	Polyester film base was introduced.
1960s	Panoramic x-ray machines were marketed.
1966	A recessed long-beam tube head was introduced. Further to this, there was no considerable development in the design of the x-ray equipment.
1968	International Association of Dento-Maxillofacial Radiology was formed.

Chapter **2**

Radiation Physics

- *Introduction*
- *Ionizing Radiation (Particulate Radiation and Electromagnetic Radiation)*
- *X-radiation*
    Properties of X-rays
- *X-ray Production*
- *X-ray Tube*
- *Electricity/Electric Current and Circuits*
- *Transformers*
- *Working of the X-ray Tube*
- *Types of Radiation*
- *Factors Controlling the X-ray Beam*
- *Quality of the X-ray Beam*
- *Quantity of the X-ray Beam*
- *Half-value Layer*

There is a single light of science, and to brighten it anywhere is to brighten it everywhere.

– Isaac Asimov

A neutron walked into a bar and asked how much for a drink.
The bartender replied,
"for you, no charge."

– Jaime - Internet Chemistry Jokes

By convention there is colour,
by convention sweetness,
by convention bitterness,
but in reality there are atoms and space.

– Democritus (400 BC)

INTRODUCTION

'Matter' is anything that occupies space and has mass. 'Energy' results when the state of matter is altered. The fundamental unit of matter is the atom. The atoms can be described as the basic building blocks of matter.

The atom consists of a central nucleus and orbiting electrons (Fig. 2-1). An atom is identified by the composition of its nucleus and the arrangement of its orbiting electrons.

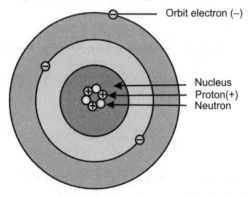

Fig. 2-1: Structure of an atom

The nucleus is composed of protons and neutrons. The protons and neutrons are collectively called as nucleons. The protons carry positive electrical charge and the neutrons are electrically neutral. The number of protons and neutrons in the nucleus of an atom determines its atomic weight. The number of protons is the same as the number of orbiting electrons and determines the atomic number. Hydrogen has an atomic number of 1 and hahnium (Hn) has an atomic number of 105.

Electrons are tiny negatively charged particles with negligible mass. Its weight is 1/1800 as much as a proton or neutron. The electrons travel around the nucleus in orbits or shells. An atom can have a maximum of seven shells (K, L, M, N, O, P, and Q). These shells represent different energy levels. The number of electrons (Fig. 2-2) each shell can hold is given below.

Shell	Number of electrons
K	2
L	8
M	18
N	32
O	50
P	72
Q	98

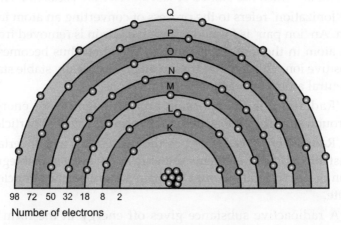

98 72 50 32 18 8 2

Number of electrons

Fig. 2-2: Electrons in the shell

The electrons are held in place in the orbit by the electrostatic force (binding energy or binding force) between the positive nucleus and the negative electrons. The distance between the nucleus and the orbiting electrons determines the binding energy. The electrons in the K shell have a greater binding energy than the electrons in the outer shell. This binding energy is measured in electron-volts (eV) or kilo-electron-volts (keV).

1 keV=1000 eV

The atoms can combine with each other to form molecules. A molecule is the smallest amount of a substance with distinct characteristic properties. In a molecule the atoms are joined by chemical bonds. Molecules are formed by either the transfer of electrons or by sharing the electrons between the outermost shells of atoms.

The atoms can exist in a neutral or in an electrically unbalanced state. An atom is referred to as a neutral atom when it contains equal number of protons and electrons.

An atom with incompletely filled outer shell is electrically unbalanced and tries to gain electron to achieve a stable state. If an atom gains an electron it will have more negative charge. If an atom loses an electron it will have more positive charge. An atom, which has gained or lost an electron, is called an ion.

'Ionization' refers to the process of converting an atom into ion. An 'ion pair' is formed when an electron is removed from an atom in the ionization process. The atom thus becomes a positive ion. This ion pair tries to attain electrically stable state (neutral atom) by reacting with other ions.

'Radiation' is the emission and propagation of energy through space or a substance in the form of waves or particles.

'Radioactivity' is defined as the process by which certain unstable atoms or elements undergo spontaneous disintegration or decay, in an attempt to attain a more balanced nuclear state.

A radioactive substance gives off energy in the form of particles or rays as a result of the disintegration of atomic nuclei.

IONIZING RADIATION

Ionizing radiation is defined as radiation that is capable of producing ions by removing or adding electron to an atom. Ionizing radiation is grouped into the following:
a. Particulate radiation
b. Electromagnetic radiation.

Particulate Radiation

Particulate radiations are tiny particles of matter possessing mass and traveling in straight lines and at high speeds. There are four recognized types of particulate radiation. These are described below.

Electrons are the beta particles or cathode rays. Beta particles are fast-moving electrons emitted from the nucleus of radioactive atoms. Cathode rays are high-speed electrons originating in an x-ray tube.

Alpha particles are emitted from the nucleus of heavy metals and exist as two protons and neutrons, without any electrons.

Protons are accelerated particles, specifically hydrogen nuclei, with a mass of 1 and a charge of +1.

Neutrons are accelerated particles with a mass of 1 and without any electrical charge.

Electromagnetic Radiation

Electromagnetic radiation is defined as the propagation of wave-like energy (without mass) through space or matter. Electromagnetic radiations are either man-made (artificial) or natural. These radiations are the following:

• Cosmic rays
• Gamma rays
• X-rays
• Ultraviolet (U-V) rays
• Visible light
• Infrared light
• Radar waves
• Microwaves and
• Radiowaves.

When the electromagnetic radiations are grouped according to their energies it is called as the electromagnetic spectrum (Fig. 2-3). The individual radiations of the spectrum differ in their wavelengths and frequencies and also in properties. The waves with shorter wavelengths and higher frequencies have more photon energy.

The energy waves have a crest (height of the wave) and trough (depth of the wave). The distance from one crest to another is called the wavelength (λ or lambda). Figure 2-4 represents the crest and trough. The frequency of a wave refers to the number of oscillations per unit of time. The wavelength of x-rays is very short and is measured in angstrom (Å) units. Ten billion angstroms equal 1 meter.

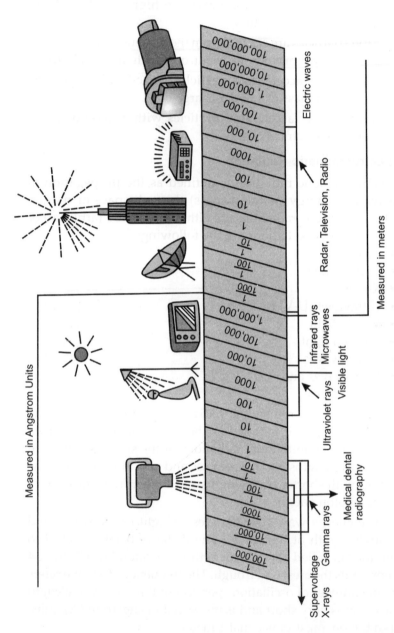

Fig. 2-3: Electromagnetic spectrum

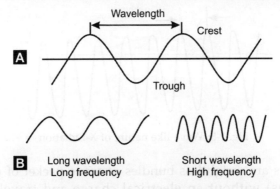

Figs 2-4A and B: (A) Crest, trough and wavelength
(B) Long wavelength and short wavelength

Angstrom is named after the 19th century Swedish physicist Anders Jonas Angstrom. 1 Å = 1/100,000,000 of a centimeter or 10^{-18} cm. The x-rays differ from visible light in the wavelength. If the wavelength is less, the frequency is more and more energy it bears. Possession of greater energy facilitates penetration of matter.

The effects of electromagnetic radiation on human tissues can be summarized as given below:
- Television and radiowaves: No effect on human tissues.
- Microwaves (low energy radiation): May produce heat within organic tissue.
- Low energy radiation capable of causing less ionization: As these have low ionization effects on living tissues, they are used in magnetic resonance imaging (MRI). This type of radiation is located near the radiowaves.
- Gamma rays and X-rays: These rays are capable of causing ionization.

X-RADIATION

X-radiation is a high-energy, ionizing electromagnetic radiation. X-rays have properties of being both waves and particles (particles or photons are bundles of energy without any mass or weight and traveling as waves) (Fig. 2-5).

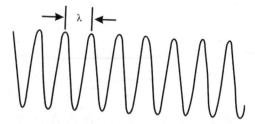

Fig. 2-5: Wave-like nature of X-radiation

X-rays are weightless bundles or wave packet of energy (photons) without an electrical charge and traveling in waveform with a specific frequency at the speed of light. A photon is equivalent to one quantum of energy. The x-ray beam is made up of millions of individual photons.

Properties of X-rays

- X-rays are invisible and cannot be detected by any of the human senses
- X-rays have no mass or weight
- X-rays have no charge
- X-rays travel in the same speed as light (186,000 miles/second)
- X-rays travel as waves and have short wavelength
- X-rays have a high frequency
- X-rays travel in straight lines and can be deflected or scattered
- X-rays diverge from the source
- X-rays cannot be focused to a point
- X-rays have penetrating power
- X-rays are absorbed by matter. The absorption depends on the atomic structure of matter and the wavelength of the x-rays
- X-rays cause ionization of matter
- X-rays can cause certain substances to fluoresce or emit radiation in longer wavelength
- X-rays can produce image on photographic film
- X-rays can cause biologic changes in living cells

- An electrical and magnetic fields fluctuate perpendicular to the direction of x-rays and at right angles to each other (Fig. 2-6).

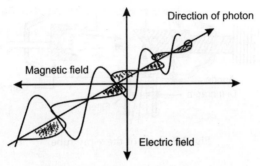

Fig. 2-6: Electrical and magnetic fields

X-RAY PRODUCTION

X-rays are produced when high-speed electrons collide with a positively charged target. This is the fundamental principle of x-ray production.

X-RAY TUBE (FIG. 2-7)

The x-ray tube is made up of borosilicate glass vacuum tube. The component parts of the x-ray tube are the following:
- A leaded-glass housing
- A negative electrode (cathode)
- A positive electrode (anode)

The glass tube is a vacuum tube. Evacuation of the glass tube is done to prevent the loss of kinetic energy of the electrons by colliding with the gas molecules and also to prevent the oxidation burn out of the filament. The central area of the x-ray tube has an opening (window) that permits the x-ray beam to exit.

The cathode consists of a tungsten wire filament, which is 1 inch long and 0.2 cm in diameter. The filament present in the cathode is the source of electrons when heated to incandescence. The cathode also contains a molybdenum-focusing cup, which

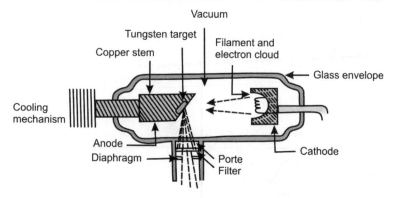

Fig. 2-7: Parts of the x-ray tube

electrostatically focuses the electrons on to the tungsten target of the anode.

The anode consists of a thin tungsten plate embedded in a solid copper block. Tungsten is used as a target material because of the following reasons:
- Its high atomic number (74)
- High melting point (3370°C)
- Low vapor pressure.

The target converts the bombarding electrons into x-ray photons.

The sharpness of the radiographic image improves if the focal spot in the target is small. Focal spot is the area where the beam of electrons from the filament is directed. The target is placed at an angle of 20° with respect to the central beam to achieve a small focal spot and to effectively distribute the striking electrons for better heat dissipation.

LINE FOCUS PRINCIPLE

The effective focal spot (the focal spot perpendicular to the electron beam) is smaller (about 1×1 mm) than the actual focal spot (the focal spot projected perpendicular from the target), which is about 1×3 mm. This principle is called as the line focus principle.

HEEL EFFECT

Heel effect refers to the loss of intensity of x-ray beam in the peripheral region (Fig. 2-8). The cathode side of the beam is more intense than the anode side. This is due to self-absorption of some of the bremsstrahlung photons by the target.

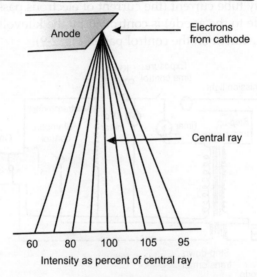

Fig. 2-8: Heel effect

When the kinetic energy of the stream of electrons originating in the cathode is directed at the target, about 99% of the kinetic energy is converted into heat and only 1% is utilized for the production of x-rays. Hence, there must be a mechanism by which the excess heat produced can be dissipated. The copper black is used to dissipate the excessive heat produced as the target is placed within the copper black and copper is a good conductor of heat. The other methods for dissipating the excess heat are:

- Use of rotating anode in which the stream of electrons would strike at different locations of the anode
- Insulating oil around the tube
- Angulating the target
- Air-conditioning of the x-ray room.

ELECTRICITY/ELECTRIC CURRENT AND CIRCUITS

The milliamperage (mA) is the measurement of the number of electrons moving through the filament. The number of electrons passing through the cathode filament can be controlled by mA adjustment on the control panel of the x-ray machine. The voltage of the x-ray tube current (the current of electrons passing from the cathode to the anode) is controlled by the kilovoltage peak (kVp) adjustment on the control panel (Fig. 2-9).

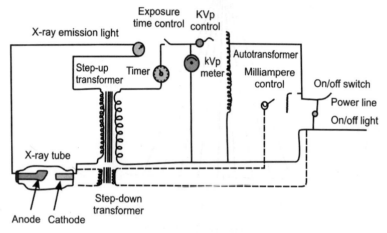

Fig. 2-9: Electrical circuit of x-ray tube

The two circuits used in the production of x-rays are a low-voltage filament circuit and a high voltage circuit. The filament circuit uses 7 to 10 volts and is controlled by the milliamperage settings. The high-voltage circuit uses 65 to 70 kVp and provides high voltage required to accelerate the electrons as they move from the cathode to the anode and to generate x-rays in the x-ray tube. The kVp is controlled by the kilovoltage settings of the x-ray machine.

TRANSFORMERS (FIG. 2-10)

A transformer either increases or decreases the voltage in an electrical circuit. A step-down transformer is used to decrease the voltage from the incoming 110 or 220-line voltage to 7 to 10

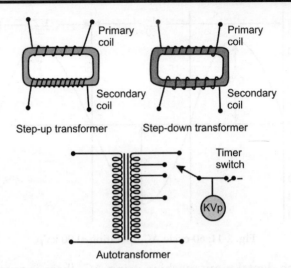

Fig. 2-10: Different transformers used in the x-ray machine

volts. The step-down transformer has more wire coils in the primary coil or input coil (it receives the alternating electrical current) than in the secondary coil or output coil. The electrical current that energizes the primary coil induces a current in the secondary coil. A step-up transformer is used to increase the voltage from the incoming 110 or 220-line voltage to 65 to 70 kVp. It has more wire coils in the secondary coil than the primary coil.

An autotransformer serves as a voltage compensator for correcting any minor fluctuation in the current.

The electric current can either be alternating current (AC) or direct current (DC). DC refers to current flowing in one direction only in an electric circuit, whereas AC flows in one direction and then flows in the opposite direction in the circuit. In the dental x-ray machine with AC circuit, during the reversal of the direction of the current, x-rays are not produced.

The term cycle in AC is the flow of current in one direction and then the reversal and current flow in the opposite direction. There are usually 60 cycles per second in most AC circuits (Fig. 2-11).

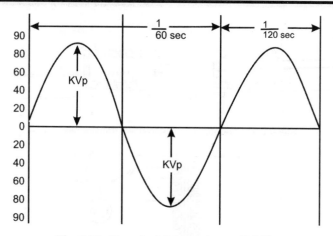

Fig. 2-11: 60-cycle AC operating at 90 kVp

In the dental x-ray machine using AC, there is reversal of polarity in the x-ray tube 60 times per second when the direction of the current is reversed, the tungsten filament becomes the positive pole and the tungsten target becomes the negative pole. During the alternating 1/120 second (half of a cycle) when the current is reversed, x-rays are not produced as there is no movement of electrons to the target from the filament or in other words there is a blockage of current from traveling across the tube. Countering this reversal is called rectification (Fig. 2-12). As the dental x-ray tube is designed to produce this

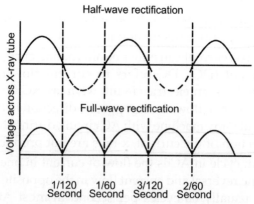

Fig. 2-12: Half-wave and full-wave rectification

effect, it is said to be self or half-wave rectified. In full-wave rectification or full wave rectified circuit, even the negative half of the cycle is used for the production of x-rays. In these machines, x-rays are not produced in pulses but as a stream of x-rays.

WORKING OF THE X-RAY TUBE

When the tungsten filament in the cathode is heated to incandescence or red hot, thermionic emission occurs. Thermionic emission is the release of electrons from the tungsten filament when the electric current passes through it and heats it up. The electrons present in the outer shell of the tungsten atom acquire sufficient energy to detach from the filament surface resulting in the formation of an electron cloud around the filament.

When the high-voltage circuit is activated, the electrons produced at the cathode are accelerated across the x-ray tube to the anode. The negatively charged molybdenum focusing cup electrostatically focuses the stream of electrons on to the target.

As the electrons travel from the cathode to the anode, their kinetic energy is suddenly arrested by the collision with the tungsten target and thus x-rays are produced. However, it must be emphasized that about 99% of the kinetic energy of the electrons will be converted into heat and only 1% will be utilized for the production of x-rays.

The exposure time is the duration of time when x-rays are produced. Apart from the mA and kVp adjustments, it is possible to adjust the exposure time also. The timing control device controls the exposure time. It completes the circuit with the high-voltage transformer. This controls the time during which high voltage is applied across the x-ray tube.

The x-ray tube does not emit a continuous stream of radiation, but a series of impulses of radiation. The number of impulses depends on the number of cycles per second in the electric current used. In 60-cycle alternating current, there are

60 pulses of x-rays per second. Each impulse lasts only 1/120 second as no x-rays are emitted in the negative half of the cycle when the polarity of the tube is reversed. A full-wave rectified x-ray machine produces 120 bursts of x-ray photons per second.

TYPES OF RADIATION (FIG. 2-13)

The two types of x-radiations produced in the x-ray tube are:
1. Bremsstrahlung radiation
2. Characteristic radiation.

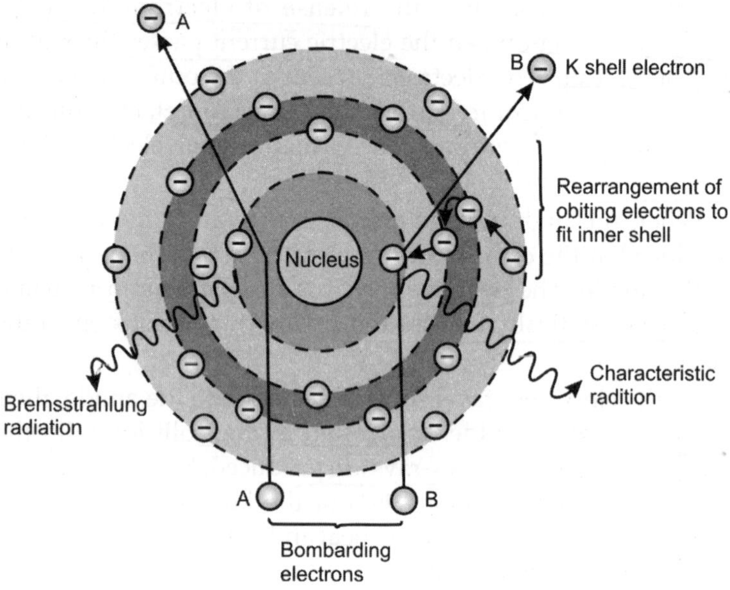

Fig. 2-13: Bremsstrahlung and characteristic radiations
(diagrammatic representation)

Bremsstrahlung Radiation

The word bremsstrahlung radiation originates from the German word for "braking radiation" . When a stream of electrons is directed towards the target, there can be two possibilities.

The first possibility is rare in which the high-speed electron may hit the nucleus of the tungsten atom, resulting in loss of all its energy. The second possibility is, the electron does not hit the nucleus. As shown in the diagram, the entering high-speed electron, (A) may be slowed down and veered off in its course by the positive pull of the nucleus. In the slowing process, the loss of energy is given off as x-rays and heat. This is the origin of bremsstrahlung radiation. Since the tungsten atom is not a single one, the bremsstrahlung radiation is repeated for an infinite number of times. The exiting electron will enter another tungsten atom and the process will be repeated with the production of more x-rays. Bremsstrahlung radiation is the main source of x-ray production in the x-ray tube.

Characteristic Radiation

If the entering high-speed electron, B possesses greater energy, it may hit and dislodge one of the orbiting electrons of the tungsten atom. This depends on the energy of the high-speed electron, which should be more than the binding energy of the orbital electron. When the orbiting electron is dislodged, a rearrangement or cascading of electrons inward fills up the electron vacancies in the inner shells. This rearrangement produces a loss of energy that is expressed as x-ray energy. These x-rays are called characteristic x-rays and account for only a very small part of the total x-rays generated. This type of x-rays is produced in x-ray machines using a higher operating voltage (70 kVp or more).

FACTORS CONTROLLING THE X-RAY BEAM

There are various factors controlling the quality and quantity of the x-rays. These factors can be modified to suit the requirement in practice.

Tube Voltage

As the kilo voltage peak (kVp) is increased, the energy of each electron striking the target increases. This results in increase in the number of x-ray photons generated, increases the mean energy of the photons or enhances the penetrating power of the x-ray photons, and increases the maximum energy of the photons. As the kVp is increased, the contrast of the resultant radiographic image becomes less. Therefore, kVp should not be increased beyond the optimum level.

Tube Current

The tube current (mA) determines the number of x-ray photons generated. As the mA is increased, more number of electrons is generated at the cathode, which strike the target to produce more number of x-ray photons. But in practice, the quantity of x-ray photons generated depends on the mA as well as on the duration of time the x-ray machine is operated and is expressed as the product of tube current and time (mAs).

Quantity of x-rays generated = milliamperage (mA) × exposure time in seconds (s)

Exposure Time

When the exposure time is doubled by keeping both the mA and kVp constant, the number of x-ray photons generated also doubles. Thus changing the exposure time influences the quantity of x-rays produced or greater the exposure time, greater will be the amount of x-rays produced.

Filtration

An x-ray beam consists of x-ray photons of different energy (polychromatic spectrum). Only those photons with sufficient energy can penetrate structures to cast image. X-ray photons with less penetrating power will be absorbed by the soft tissues and do not contribute to image formation. Thus, these x-ray photons cause unnecessary radiation exposure to the patient.

Filtration is the process of removing x-ray photons of less penetrating power by placing aluminium disks in the path of the primary beam which allow only x-ray photons with sufficient energy to pass through.

A filter is a device made up of an aluminium disk placed in the path of the primary x-ray beam to absorb x-ray photons of less penetrating power.

Filtration is of three types:
a. Inherent filtration
b. Added filtration
c. Total filtration.

Inherent filtration is produced by materials, which the x-ray beam encounters as it leaves from the target. These materials are the glass wall of the x-ray tube, insulating oil present around the tube, and the barrier material, which prevents the oil from leaking out. The inherent filtration usually provides 0.5 to 2.0 mm aluminium equivalent of filtration.

Added filtration refers to any additional aluminium disk placed in the path of the primary beam.

Total filtration refers to the sum of inherent and added filtration. The total filtration should be equal to the equivalent of 1.5 mm of aluminium up to 70 kVp and 2.5 mm of aluminium above 70 kVp.

Collimation

When a patient is exposed to a beam of radiation, the patient's tissues absorb 90% of the x-ray photons and only 10% will be utilized for the production of the image. Most of these absorbed photons are the source of scattered photons, which travel in different directions and cause film fog. The absorbed photons are usually from the peripheral portion of the x-ray beam.

Collimation is the process of restriction of the size of the x-ray beam and thus the volume of the irradiated tissue of the patient from which the scattered photons originate.

Collimator (Fig. 2-14) is a device that is used to shape or restrict the size of the x-ray beam striking the patient's tissues.

Collimation has the following uses:
• It decreases the size of the x-ray beam
• It decreases the volume of the irradiated tissues of the patient and thus decreases the radiation exposure

- It decreases the amount of scattered photons generated
- It minimizes the film fog and enhances the image quality.

The collimator is made up of a material such as lead, which is capable of absorbing the radiation. Various collimators used in dental radiography are the diaphragm, tubular, and rectangular collimators (Figs 2-14A to D).

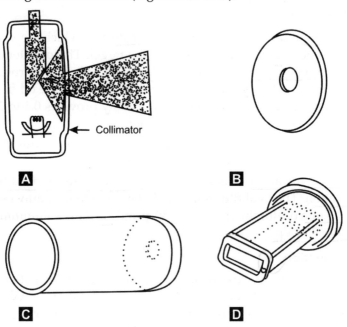

Figs 2-14A to D: Different collimators used in dental radiography. (A) Collimator reduces the size of the x-ray beam (B) Diaphragm collimator (C) Tubular collimator (D) Rectangular collimator.

The diaphragm collimator is a disk made up of lead having an aperture in the center. It usually has a thickness of 1/16 of an inch. This is placed between the target and the window of the x-ray tube. Window of the x-ray tube is the opening through which the beam of x-rays come out of the tube.

The tubular collimator is a tube lined with or constructed of a radiopaque material. This is used along with the diaphragm collimator at one end. The rectangular collimator helps in defining the x-ray beam to a size larger than the size of the film.

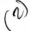 **Inverse Square Law**

Inverse square law states that the intensity of an x-ray beam at a given point (number of x-ray photons per cross-sectional area per unit time) is inversely proportional to the square of the distance from the source of radiation. Diagrammatic representation of inverse square law is shown in Figure 2-15.

The mathematical formula used to calculate inverse square law is given below:

$$\frac{\text{Original intensity } (I_1)}{\text{New intensity } (I_2)} = \frac{\text{New distance}^2 \ (D_2)^2}{\text{Original distance}^2 \ (D_1)^2}$$

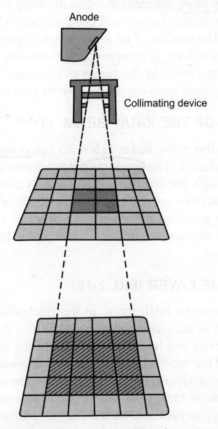

Fig. 2-15: Diagrammatic representation of inverse square law

The reason for this decrease in the intensity of the x-ray beam is due to the divergent nature of the x-rays from the source. Thus, if the distance from the source to the object is increased, the intensity of the x-ray beam decreases, thereby changing the image quality. If the distance from the source to the film is doubled (e.g. from 8 inches to 16 inches), it results in a beam that is one-fourth as intense.

QUALITY OF THE X-RAY BEAM   *Tube voltage*

The quality of the x-ray beam refers to its mean energy or penetrating ability. X-rays with shorter wavelengths have more penetrating power, whereas those with longer wavelengths have less penetrating power and get absorbed by the patient's soft tissues. The quality of an x-ray beam is governed by the kVp. When the kVp is increased, the velocity of electrons (kinetic energy) striking the target is increased. It results in x-ray photons with high energy and better penetrating power.

QUANTITY OF THE X-RAY BEAM   *Tube current*

Quantity of the x-ray beam refers to the number of x-ray photons produced. The amperage determines the electrons passing through the filament. When mA is increased, more number of electrons are released in the cathode and they strike the target to produce more number of x-ray photons. The quantity depends on the product of mA and exposure time in seconds (mAs).

HALF-VALUE LAYER (FIG. 2-16)

Half-value layer or HVL refers to the thickness of specified material such as aluminium required to reduce the intensity of an x-ray beam by one-half. The thickness of any given material where 50% of the incident energy has been attenuated is known as the half-value layer (HVL). The HVL is expressed in units of distance (mm or cm). Like the attenuation coefficient, it is photon energy dependant. Increasing the penetrating energy of a stream of photons will result in an increase in a material's

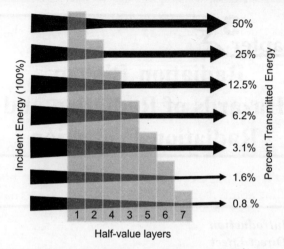

Fig. 2-16: Diagrammatic representation of half-value layer

HVL. The HVL is often used in radiography simply because it is easier to remember values and perform simple calculations. In a shielding calculation, such as illustrated below, it can be seen that if the thickness of one HVL is known, it is possible to quickly determine how much material is needed to reduce the intensity to less than 1%.

Chapter 3

Radiation Biology, Hazards of Radiation and Radiation Protection

- *Introduction*
- *Direct Effect*
- *Indirect Effect*
    Radiation Injury
    Effects of Radiation
- *Units of Measurement of Radiation*
- *Hazards of Radiation*
    Sources of Radiation Exposure
    Radiation-induced Changes in Biologic Molecules
- *Dosimetry*
- *Radiation Protection*

The Saddest Aspect of Life Right Now is That Science Gathers Knowledge Faster than Society Gathers Wisdom.

– **Isaac Asimov**

INTRODUCTION

Radiation biology is the study of the effects of ionizing radiation on living tissue. The ionizing radiations are harmful and produce biologic changes in living tissues. X-rays are a form of ionizing radiation.

The cell damage caused by x-rays is mainly due to the formation of free radicals. As the x-ray photons strike the living cells, there is ionization of water resulting in the formation of hydrogen and hydroxyl free radicals (radiolysis of water) (Fig. 3-1).

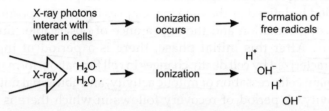

Fig. 3-1: Radiolysis of water and formation of free radicals

The free radicals are unstable and highly reactive. The lifetime of a free radical is about 10^{-10} seconds. The free radicals attain stability either by:

1. Combining without causing any changes in the molecule
2. Combining with other free radicals to cause changes
3. Combining with ordinary molecules to form toxic substances (e.g. hydrogen peroxide).

Damage to living tissues may be either due to the direct effect or due to the indirect effect.

DIRECT EFFECT

In the direct effect, there is alteration of biologic molecules when the x-ray photons directly strike the cells. The affected molecules become structurally and functionally different from the original molecules. Direct injuries from radiation exposure are relatively rare.

INDIRECT EFFECT

Indirect effects of radiation are due to the formation of free radicals, which combine to form toxins and not because of a direct hit by x-ray photons. The indirect effects are due to high water content of the cells. The x-ray photons are absorbed by water within a cell, resulting in free radical formation. These free radicals combine to form toxins such as hydrogen peroxide (H_2O_2).

Radiation Injury

Following radiation exposure, there is a latent period. The latent period is defined as the time that elapses between exposure to ionizing radiation and the appearance of observable clinical signs. After this initial phase, there is a period of injury characterized by cell death, changes in cell formation, formation of giant cells, cessation of mitotic activity, and abnormal mitotic activity. A period of recovery follows in which there is cell repair. The additive effects of radiation are due to the accumulation of unrepaired cells within the tissues. This is called the cumulative effects of radiation.

Factors Influencing Radiation Injury

Total Dose

Total dose refers to the amount of radiation energy absorbed.

Dose Rate

Dose rate is the rate at which exposure to radiation occurs and absorption takes place (dose rate = dose/time). High dose rate results in more radiation damage as there is no sufficient time for the cellular damage to be repaired.

Amount of Tissue Irradiated

Amount of tissue irradiated refers to the areas of the body exposed to radiation. Total body irradiation results in more systemic effects than when a small, localized area is exposed to radiation.

Sensitivity of Cells

More serious damage occurs in cells that are most sensitive to radiation (e.g. rapidly dividing and young cells).

Age

Age is an important factor in radiation injury. Children are more prone to radiation damage than adults.

Effects of Radiation

Short-term Effects

Short-term effects of radiation refer to the damage occurring within minutes, days, or weeks. Short-term effects are due to large amounts of radiation absorbed in a short period of time as in nuclear accidents or atomic bomb explosions. Acute radiation syndrome (ARS) is a short-term effect characterized by nausea, vomiting, diarrhea, loss of hair and hemorrhage. Table 3-1 shows classification of tissues based on their sensitivity.

Long-term Effects

Long-term effects appear in years, decades, or generation after radiation exposure. The long-term effects are due to small amounts of radiation absorbed repeatedly over a long period of time. The long-term effects vary from induction of carcinoma to genetic effects. Table 3-2 shows different tissues or organs and radiation effect.

Somatic and Genetic Effects

Somatic effects are radiation effects seen in body cells other than reproductive cells.

Some of the somatic effects of radiation are induction of cancer, leukemia and cataract.

Genetic effects are seen in the reproductive cells and are not manifested in the individual exposed to radiation, but are passed on to future generations. Genetic damage cannot be repaired.

Table 3-1: Radiation sensitivity of different tissues

* **High sensitivity**
  - Lymphoid organ
  - Bone marrow
  - Testes
  - Intestines
* **Intermediate sensitivity**
  - Fine vasculature
  - Growing cartilage
  - Growing bone
* **Low sensitivity**
  - Salivary glands
  - Lungs
  - Kidney
  - Liver
  - Optic lens

Table 3-2: Different tissues and radiation effects

Tissue or organ	Radiation effect
Hematopoietic	Leukemia
Reproductive	Mutations
Thyroid	Carcinoma
Skin	Carcinoma
Eyes	Cataract

UNITS OF MEASUREMENT OF RADIATION

Exposure

Exposure refers to the measurement of ionization in air produced by x-rays. The unit of exposure is roentgen (R). One 'R' is the quantity of x-radiation or gamma radiation that produces an electrical charge of 2.58×10^{-4} coulombs in a kilogram of air at standard temperature and pressure (STP). It is also defined as the amount of x- or gamma-radiation that will produce in 1 cc of air (STP) 2.08×10^9 ion pairs. The R is used to measure the intensity of radiation to which an object is exposed. In SI system, exposure is measured in coulombs per kilogram (C/kg).

$1 R = 2.58 \times 10^{-4}$ C/kg and 1 C/kg = 3.88×10^3 R

Absorbed Dose

Absorbed dose is the amount of energy absorbed by a tissue. Radiation absorbed dose or *rad* is the unit of dose. Rad is a special unit of absorbed dose that is equal to the deposition of 100 ergs of energy per gram of tissue (100 ergs/g). In SI system, the unit of measurement of dose is Gray (Gy).

1 Gy = 1 joule/kg or 100 rads

1 rad = 100 ergs/g of absorber or 0.01 Gy

Dose Equivalent

Dose equivalent measurement is used to compare the biologic effects of different types of radiation. The traditional unit of dose-equivalent is the *rem* (roentgen equivalent-man). Rem is the product of absorbed dose (rad) and a quality factor specific for the type of radiation. In SI system, the unit of dose-equivalent is the Sievert (Sv).

1 rem = 0.01 Sv and 1 Sv = 100 rems

Quality Factor

Quality factor (Q) of radiation refers to its biologic effect relative to standard exposure of x-ray. A dose of 0.1 Gy caused by fast neutrons has the same biologic effect as 1.0 Gy of x-rays. Therefore, the Q of fast neutrons is 10 (1.0/0.1 = 10).

Relative Biological Effectiveness

Relative biological effectiveness (RBE) is similar to quality factor, but refers to laboratory investigations.

Radioactivity

Radioactivity refers to the decay rate of a sample of radioactive material. The traditional unit of radioactivity is the curie (Ci) and in SI system the unit is the Becquerel (Bq). Ci corresponds to the activity of l g of radium (3.7×10^{10} disintegrations/second).

1 mCi = 37 mega Bq and 1 Bq = 2.7×10^{-11} Ci

HAZARDS OF RADIATION

Sources of Radiation Exposure

Radiation exposure may be due to a variety of radiation sources (Table 3-3).

Natural Radiation (Background Radiation)

Naturally occurring radiations are cosmic radiation and terrestrial radiation. Cosmic radiations are subatomic particles and photons of extraterrestrial origin (primary cosmic radiation) and particles and photons produced by the interaction of primary cosmic radiation with atoms and molecules of the atmosphere of earth (secondary cosmic radiation). Terrestrial radiation exposure is due to naturally occurring radioactive substances such as radium, uranium, and thorium with their decay products and potassium-40. Various building materials used can also contribute to radiation exposure. Apart from the cosmic radiation and terrestrial radiation, there are internal sources that are taken up from the external environment by inhalation and ingestion.

Man-made Radiation

The sources of man-made radiations are diagnostic radiography, therapeutic use of ionizing radiations, consumer and industrial products (coal-fired electric plants, pocket watches, tobacco products, smoke alarm, cellular phone, etc.), airline travel, atomic fall-outs, and nuclear accidents. Table 3-3 shows various radiation sources and approximate exposure.

Table 3-3: Various radiation sources and approximate exposure

Radiation Sources	Whole Body (mrem/year)
Natural	
Radon	200.00
Cosmic	27.00
Terrestrial	28.00
Internal	39.00
Artificial	
Medical or dental x-rays	53.00
Consumer products	9.00
Other sources	
Occupational	Less than 1.00
Nuclear fuel cycle	Less than 1.00
Fall-out	Less than 1.0

Radiation-induced Changes In Biologic Molecules

Proteins

Radiation exposure to the proteins can cause structural alterations leading to denaturation. There can also be inter- and intramolecular crosslinking. The inactivation of enzyme molecule can result in functional failure of biological reactions.

Nucleic Acids

Deoxyribonucleic acid (DNA) is more sensitive to radiation than ribonucleic acid (RNA). Radiation can result in chemical disruption of the DNA molecules.

Cells

Radiation can induce structural and functional changes in cellular organelles that culminate in cell death. The nucleus of a cell is more sensitive to radiation than the cytoplasm. There can be cell division arrest. Radiation affects the DNA and chromosomes of the nucleus. Radiation has harmful effects on chromosomes, causing chromosomal aberrations.

Chromosome Aberrations

Chromosome aberrations are more marked at the time of mitosis when the DNA condenses. Higher doses are required for cytoplasmic changes to take place. These changes are permeability and structural changes. Vegetative intermitotic cells are more radiosensitive.

Irradiation can also result in mitotic delay of dividing cells.

Oral Cavity

The oral changes due to radiation are mainly the result of radiotherapy for malignant lesions. As the oral mucous membrane contains radiosensitive, vegetative and differentiating intermitotic cells in the basal layer, marked redness and inflammation (mucositis) are seen by the end of second week of radiotherapy. Secondary infection (candidiasis), caused by *Candida albicans* is a complication of radiation mucositis.

Taste Buds

Changes in the taste buds are extensive degeneration of normal histologic pattern. There can also be loss of taste sensation in the second or third week of radiotherapy.

Salivary Glands

The salivary glands are exposed to radiation during radiotherapy of the head and neck region. The parenchymal cells are more radiosensitive. There can be inflammatory response involving serous acini, increase in serum amylase, and progressive fibrosis; adiposis; loss of fine vasculature, and parenchymal degeneration. Saliva flow is diminished and it becomes more viscous. The pH of the saliva also decreases (becomes acidic).

Teeth

Though the mineralized tissues of teeth are resistant to radiation, the pulp tissue exhibits fibroatrophy. Irradiation during the developmental stage of dentition can result in growth retardation of teeth. Irradiation can also result in malformation of teeth. Radiation caries is a rampant type of dental caries that occurs due to radiotherapy involving the head and neck region for treatment of cancer. This is secondary to changes seen in the salivary glands and saliva such as the following:

• Reduced flow rate
• Decrease in pH (salivary pH becomes more acidic)
• Lack of buffering capacity of saliva
• Increased viscosity.

Lack of normal cleansing action of the saliva results in the accumulation of local irritants that can cause increased incidence of dental caries in the postirradiation period.

Bone

The effects of radiation are more marked in the mandible. The initial change is seen in the vasculature. The bone marrow becomes hypoxic and hypocellular. There are atrophic changes within the bone, eventually leading to necrotic changes (osteoradionecrosis). This usually follows any trauma such as dental extraction carried out in an irradiated patient and subsequent infection of the socket due to decreased healing potential of the bone as a result of improper blood supply. Osteoradionecrosis occurs due to decreased capacity of the bone to resist infection.

Osteoradionecrosis (ORN) is defined as exposed irradiated bone that fails to heal over a period of three months (Fig. 3-2). The incidence of ORN is approximately about 10–15% following radiotherapy. The initial findings associated with ORN are the following:

• Foul odor
• Exposed necrotic bone

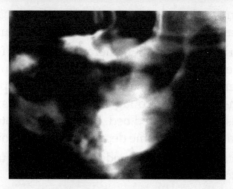

Fig. 3-2: Radiographic appearance of ORN

- Severe pain
- Discharging fistulae
- Mucosal defect

Prior to beginning radiation therapy, all patients should undergo a thorough dental evaluation, including full mouth radiographs, dental and periodontal assessment and prognosis for each tooth. Outline a complete treatment plan, taking into account the patient's motivation and compliance based upon discussions with the patient and his or her family. Patient education regarding the need for meticulous oral hygiene and frequent follow-up must be stressed.

The dentist should perform prophylaxis, periodontal scaling, caries control and fabrication of fluoride trays.

Teeth that cannot be restored with conservative or endodontic therapy should be extracted. Ideally, extractions should be performed 3 weeks prior to the beginning of radiation therapy. Extraction of teeth during radiation therapy should be discouraged and delayed until the completion of treatment with resolution of the radiation mucositis.

To prevent radiation caries, patients should begin daily fluoride treatment with 1% neutral sodium fluoride gel in prefabricated trays for 5 minutes each day.

Medical therapy in treatment of ORN is primarily supportive, involving nutritional support along with superficial debridement and oral saline irrigation for local wounds. Antibiotics are indicated only for definite secondary infection.

Hyperbaric oxygen (HBO) therapy has been found to be useful in the management of ORN. HBO transiently elevates tissue oxygen tension and stimulates fibroblastic proliferation and oxygen-dependent collagen synthesis. This allows for angiogenesis in the radiated bed. This does not totally resolve the radiation injury and some degree of tissue hypoxia persists.

In some cases surgical procedures such as sequestrectomy or microvascular free tissue transfer are tried out.

DOSIMETRY

Dosimetry refers to the determination of radiation exposure or dose. Dose is the amount of energy absorbed per unit mass at a site of interest. There are various devices available for the measurement of radiation exposure.

Film Badges

As the name implies, film badges contain a film, which helps to determine the radiation exposure when processed, based on the degree of darkening. It has to be standardized with films exposed to predetermined amounts of radiation. Film in the film badges is periodically changed and sent for radiation exposure measurement (Fig. 3-3).

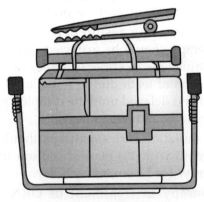

Fig. 3-3: Film badge

Ionization Chamber

An ionization chamber is used to determine the radiation exposure of a room. It consists of two oppositely charged plates, separated by a known volume of air. The plates are connected to a galvanometer to measure the charge. Before using, standard charge is applied to the plates. When the x-ray beam exposes the air, there is formation of ion pairs. The positive and negative ions get attracted to the oppositely charged plates (the positive ions to the negative plate and the negative ions to the positive plate), thus, resulting in partial discharges. Accordingly, the radiation exposure depends on the number of ion pairs produced and the drop in the potential (Fig. 3-4).

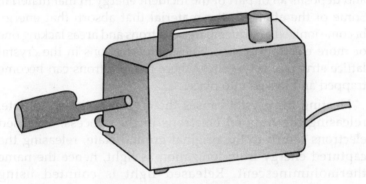

Fig. 3-4: Ionization chamber

Thermoluminescent Dosimeter

Thermoluminescent dosimeters (TLD) are based on the principle of the ability of certain crystals (e.g. lithium fluoride, LiF) to absorb the x-ray photons and generate visible light. The total light emitted is proportional to the energy absorbed by the crystal, which is measured by a photomultiplier tube. Thermoluminescent dosimeters (TLD) are often used nowadays instead of the film badges. Like a film badge, it is worn for a period of time (usually 3 months) and then processed to determine the radiation exposure. Thermoluminescent dosimeters can measure doses as low as 1 millirem, but under routine conditions their low-dose capability is approximately the same as for film badges. TLDs have a precision of approximately 15% for low doses. This precision improves to approximately 3% for high doses. The advantages of a TLD over other personnel monitors are its linearity of response to dose, its relative energy independence, and its sensitivity to low doses. It is also reusable, which is an advantage over the film badges. However, no permanent record or re-readability is provided and an immediate readout is not possible. As already stated, TLD is a phosphor, such as lithium fluoride (LiF) or calcium fluoride (CaF), in a solid crystal structure. When a TLD is exposed to ionizing radiation at ambient temperatures, the radiation interacts with the phosphor crystal and deposits all or part of the incident energy in that material. Some of the atoms in the material that absorb that energy become ionized, producing free electrons and areas lacking one or more electrons, called holes. Imperfections in the crystal lattice structure act as sites where free electrons can become trapped and locked into place.

Heating the crystal causes the crystal lattice to vibrate, releasing the trapped electrons in the process. Released electrons return to the original ground state, releasing the captured energy from ionization as light, hence the name thermoluminescent. Released light is counted using photomultiplier tubes and the number of photons counted is proportional to the quantity of radiation striking the phosphor.

Instead of reading the optical density (blackness) of a film, as is done with film badges, the amount of light released versus the heating of the individual pieces of thermoluminescent material is measured. The "glow curve" produced by this process is then related to the radiation exposure. The process can be repeated many times.

 RADIATION PROTECTION

In the previous section the harmful effects of radiation have been discussed. It is readily apparent that proper protective measures should be adopted to safeguard the individuals from the harmful effects of radiation. Though no amount of radiation is safe, as all individuals are exposed to some amount of radiation as part of diagnostic radiographic examination or accidental exposure, a maximum permissible dose (MPD) has been formulated. Radiation is associated with tissue injury even with a very low level. MPD sets a limit for radiation exposure.

MPD is defined as the maximum dose of radiation that in the light of present knowledge would not be expected to produce any significant radiation effects in the life-time of an individual.

MPD differs for nonoccupationally and occupationally exposed persons. For nonoccupationally exposed persons, the MPD is 0.005 Sv/year. For occupationally exposed persons, the MPD is calculated by using the formula,

$$MPD = (Age - 18) \times 5 \text{ rem}$$

The average permissible dose for such persons is 0.05 Sv/year. From the formula it is clear that individuals younger than 18 years of age should not be employed in the radiology department or anywhere radiation is made use of for various purposes.

The various methods adopted for radiation protection should be directed at:
• The patients on whom diagnostic radiographic examination is performed
• The operator associated with the process of radiography
• Others who are not associated with radiography.

Protection of the Patient

There are a number of mandatory steps to be followed during routine diagnostic radiographic examination. These steps are mentioned below:
• Use of good machines manufactured by reputed manu-facturing companies.
• A radiograph should be taken only if it is a must and if it is essential for arriving at a diagnosis. A radiographic examination cannot be justified unless it helps in the treatment •

- The exposure should be as minimum as possible. An important principle is ALARA or as low as reasonably achievable
- Good quality films should be used. The sensitivity of the films should be more. The most commonly used films for dental radiography are D and E speed films that are very sensitive
- Proper technique should be employed to avoid the necessity of repeating the radiographic examination
- Good consistent processing technique also helps in preventing unnecessary repetitions
- The x-ray beam should be properly collimated to prevent the scattered radiation as well as to prevent irradiation of a larger area of the patients' body
- Aluminium filters should be used to remove x-ray photons of less penetrating power that do not contribute in the image formation, but cause unnecessary radiation exposure
- The cone-shaped devices should be replaced by long, open-ended, lead-lined cylinders
- The x-ray machine should be periodically checked for any leakage
- Patients should be asked to wear lead aprons having lead content equivalent to 0.25 mm aluminium
- Use of thyroid collors will protect the thyroid gland from the harmful effects of radiation
- Patient should not be asked to hold the film in the mouth to prevent additional exposure of tissues
- Use of screen-film (intensifying screen with film) combination during extraoral radiographic examination considerably reduces the radiation exposure.

Protection of the Operator

- The operator should not hold the film in the patient's mouth during exposure
- The operator should not stabilize the x-ray machine during exposure
- The operator should not stand directly in the path of the primary radiation

- The operator should not stand near the path of the primary radiation
- The operator should preferably stand behind a lead barrier having 0.5 mm lead equivalent during exposure (Fig. 3-5)
- If a lead barrier is not available, the operator should stand 6 feet away from the primary x-ray beam in an area called the zone of maximum safety which ranges from 90° to 135° with respect to the primary x-ray beam (Fig. 3-6)
- Radiation exposure to the operator should be periodically monitored by using personnel monitoring devices or film badges
- Rotation of duties of the operator so that continuous accidental exposure is avoided.

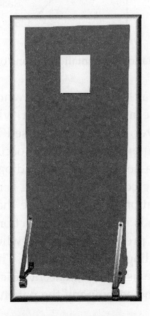

Fig. 3-5: A lead barrier

Protection of Other Persons

Generally, emphasis regarding radiation protection is made only for those who are directly involved in the radiographic

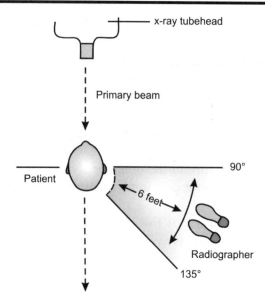

Fig. 3-6: Diagrammatic representation of zone of maximum safety

procedures such as the patients on whom the radiation exposure is made and the operator who performs the procedure. However, it must be stressed that accidental or avoidable radiation exposure can also occur to other people who are in no way associated with the radiographic procedure. As there is growing concern among the general public about the effects of radiation, it is imperative that all unnecessary radiation exposure is minimized. Protection of other persons basically refers to protection of those who are not directly involved in the radiographic procedure. This group includes even those who are using the adjacent office spaces or rooms as well as those who accompany the patients who have to be radiographed.

• Only those people whose presence is required for radiographic procedure should remain in the room
• An x-ray tube should never be directed towards the doors or doorways to avoid accidental exposure

- The walls of the room should be reinforced with barium plaster or the thickness of the walls should be increased by using an additional layer of bricks
- Caution or warning signs should be displayed
- A red light should glow when the x-ray machine is being operated, which acts as a warning signal so that nobody walks into the x-ray room
- Radiation exposure to the room should be monitored
- Radiation exposure to adjacent office premises should be monitored.

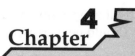

Chapter 4

Films Used in
Dental Radiography

- *Introduction*
- *Film Composition*
- *Intraoral Films*
  - *Types of Intraoral Films*
  - *Classification of Films Based on Speed*
- *Extraoral Films*
- *Duplicating Films*

We have but faith: we cannot know;
For knowledge is of things we see;
And yet we trust it comes from thee,
A beam in darkness: let it grow.

– Alfred Lord Tennyson

INTRODUCTION

The dental x-ray film serves as a recording medium or image receptor. A latent image is recorded in the x-ray film when it is exposed to information-carrying x-ray photons.

FILM COMPOSITION

The x-ray film is composed of the following components (Fig. 4-1).

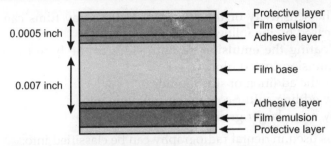

Fig. 4-1: Composition of x-ray film

Film Base

The film base is a flexible piece of polyester, having a thickness of 0.2 mm. The film base is transparent and with slight blue tint to enhance the contrast and image quality and also to provide optimal viewing conditions. The base should be able to withstand heat, moisture, and chemical exposure. The purpose of the base is to provide stable support for the emulsion and to provide adequate strength to the film.

Adhesive Layer

The adhesive layer serves to attach the film emulsion to the film base.

Film Emulsion

The film emulsion is sensitive to the x-ray photons. The emulsion consists of gelatin matrix that suspends and evenly disperses millions of microscopic silver halide crystals over the film base. During the processing, gelatin absorbs water and swells, thereby facilitating close contact and the action of chemicals with the silver halide crystals. Gelatin is derived from cattle bone.

The silver halides used in x-ray films are silver bromide (AgBr) and silver iodide (AgI). An x-ray film contains 90–99% silver bromide and only 1–10% silver iodide. The silver halide crystals absorb radiation, and the information-carrying x-ray photons produce a latent image due to the presence of these x-ray-sensitive crystals that undergo certain chemical alterations. This latent image is made visible image by processing.

The sensitivity or the efficiency of the x-ray films can be increased by the following means.

- Coating the emulsion on both sides of the base (double emulsion coated film)
- By the addition of silver iodide
- By adding sulfur-containing contaminants
- By using larger grains of silver halide.

Films used in dental radiography can be classified into:
- Intraoral films
- Extraoral films
- Duplicating films.

INTRAORAL FILMS

An intraoral film is one which is placed inside the mouth during x-ray exposure. An intraoral film is used for the visualization of the teeth and the supporting structures.

Contents of the Film Packet (Fig. 4-2)

The intraoral film is available in individual film packets. The film packet has an outer package wrapping which is made up of soft vinyl or paper. It protects the film from moisture, saliva,

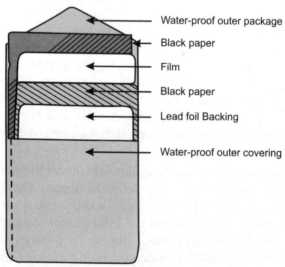

Fig. 4-2: Contents of the film packet

and light exposure. The film wrapper has two sides, tube side and label side. The tube side should always face the x-ray tube during exposure. The label side is the backside of the film packet. The tube side of the film wrapper is plane white in color with a raised embossed dot in one corner which serves in the identification of the side of the radiograph. During exposure, the embossed dot on the film must never get superimposed in the periapical region, it should be directed coronally (incisally in case of anterior teeth and occlusally in case of posterior teeth).

Within the film wrapper there is a paper film wrapper. This black paper protective sheet covers the film on either side and shields it from light exposure.

Lead foil is a single piece of thin lead foil present within the film packet and located behind the black paper between which the film is placed. This lead foil helps in preventing the back-scattered (secondary) radiation from causing film fog.

Types of Intraoral Films

Periapical Film

The periapical film is used for visualizing the entire tooth (crown and root) with an adequate area of the periapical region. Periapical films are available in three sizes.

- Size 0   It has a size of 22 × 35 mm and is used for small children
- Size 1   It has a size of 24 × 40 mm and is used for radiographing the anterior teeth in adults
- Size 2   It is the standard film used for radiographic examination. It has a size of 32 × 41 mm.

Bitewing Film

Four sizes of bitewing film are available.

- Size 0   It has a size of 22 × 35 mm and is used to examine the posterior teeth in small children
- Size 1   It has a size of 24 × 40 mm and is used to examine posterior teeth in children as well as anterior teeth in adults (when placed vertically)

- Size 2   It has a size of 32 × 41 mm and is used to examine the posterior teeth in adults
- Size 3   It has a size of 27 × 54 mm and is narrower than size 2 film. This is exclusively used for bitewing projection. This film demonstrates all the posterior teeth of one side.

Occlusal Film

The occlusal film is larger in size compared to the other intraoral films. It has a size of 57 × 76 mm. An occlusal film is used to visualize the entire arch (either the maxillary or the mandibular) in one film. This projection is also used in the localization technique to get the right angle view in conjunction with intraoral periapical radiograph. Detailed description about occlusal films is given in Chapter 9.

Classification of Films Based on Speed

Speed of an x-ray film refers to its sensitivity. A high-speed dental x-ray film requires only less amount of radiation for the image formation. Thus, use of high-speed films in the dental practice considerably reduces the exposure. Various factors responsible for increasing the sensitivity of films have already been discussed.

Based on the speed, the intraoral films are classified as A,B,C,D and E speed films. A-speed films are the slowest. B-speed and C-speed films are not used for routine intraoral radiography. D-speed (ultraspeed) and E-speed (ektaspeed) films are used for intraoral radiography. As the sensitivity of the film increases, there is a reduction in the contrast of the image. E-speed film requires only one-half the exposure time of D-speed film. Nowadays F speed films are also being marketed which are highly sensitive and contributing in the reduction of radiation exposure to the patient. However, decrease in the contrast is a major disadvantage in using F speed films. E speed films have been found to be superior in the diagnostic point of view.

EXTRAORAL FILMS

The extraoral film is one that is placed outside the mouth during exposure. These films are used when visualization of a larger area is desired.

Extraoral films used in dental radiography are available in the following sizes based on the need for visualizing the required area:

- 5 × 7 inches
- 8 × 10 inches
- 5 × 12 inches or 6 × 12 inches for panoramic radiography.

Extraoral films are usually used with intensifying screens to minimize the radiation exposure. The use of x-ray films in conjunction with the intensifying screens is referred to as screen-film combination. Nonscreen films are rarely used for extraoral radiography. Such films are called direct exposure films. A nonscreen extraoral film requires more exposure time than a screen-film combination and is not recommended for routine radiography. See also Chapter 11.

DUPLICATING FILMS

In dental radiography, duplicating film is a type of photographic film that is used to make an identical copy of an intraoral or extraoral radiograph. Duplicating film does not require exposure to x-rays. Special equipment and duplicating films are necessary for the duplication process.

Chapter 5

Grids, Intensifying Screens and Cassettes

- *Grids*
    - *Types of Grid*
- *Intensifying Screens*
    - *Composition of Intensifying Screens*
- *Cassettes*
    - *Types of Cassettes*

Yes, Heaven is thine; but this
Is a world of sweets and sours;
Our flowers are merely–flowers,
And the shadow of thy perfect bliss
Is the sunshine of ours.

– **Edgar Allan Poe**

GRIDS

When the primary radiation passes through the subject, scatter radiation is inevitably produced caused by various substances in the subject (the patient who is being radiographed). When scatter radiation reaches the film, it sensitizes even areas which should not be sensitized. This produces radiographic fog on the film without optimum contrast that is required for the optimum diagnostic quality of the radiograph. Film fog degrades the diagnostic quality of the radiograph. The x-ray grid acts as a filter, effectively removing scatter radiation before it reaches the film (the ideal name is antiscatter grid). The scattered radiation originating within the patient's tissues travel in different directions than the primary beam and causes deleterious effects in the film, as has been stated earlier, called film fog. A grid or an anti-scatter grid is used to prevent the scattered radiation from reaching the film. It should be understood that the grid does not prevent the production of scattered photons, but prevents them from reaching the film. Accordingly, the grid is positioned between the object and the film. Due to the Compton effect, it has been estimated that, the intensity of scattered photons is 2-4 times greater than the primary beam.

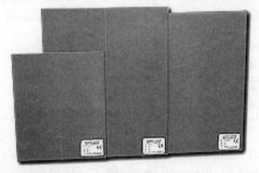

Fig. 5-1: Grids of different sizes

A grid consists of a large number of long, parallel strips of radiopaque material (e.g. lead) interspersed with radiolucent interspace material (plastic). The scattered radiation usually travels obliquely, not in the same direction as the primary x-ray beam. Hence, most of the scattered radiation gets absorbed by the lead strips of the grid. However, some of the scattered photons, which travel in the same plane as the primary beam, may contribute in the formation of the image (Fig. 5-1).

Figure 5-2 shows how the placement of grid effectively reduces the scattered radiation from reaching the film.

An ideal grid should be capable of removing 80-90% of the scattered radiation. The resultant image thus has a better contrast. This improvement in the quality is referred to as the 'contrast improvement factor (K)'.

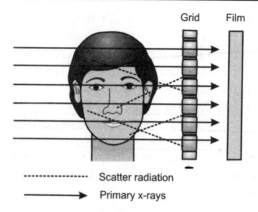

Fig. 5-2: Placement of grid effectively absorbs the scattered radiation

$$K = \frac{\text{x-ray contrast with grid}}{\text{x-ray contrast without grid}}$$

An ideal grid should have a high K value, which should be 1.5–3.5.

The total number of strips of lead in a grid varies between few hundred to thousand or more. Grids having 80 or more line pairs per inch do not show grid lines in the image.

The grid ratio (r) refers to the ratio of the thickness of the grid to the width of the radiolucent interspacer.

$$r = \frac{h}{d}$$

In the above formula, h is the thickness of the lead strips and d is their separation. The usual thickness of the lead strips is 0.005 to 0.008 cm.

Grid Density

Grid density refers to the number of x-ray absorbing strips per 1 cm. X-ray grids are available in densities of 34, 40, 60, and 80 lines per 1 cm. The higher the grid density, the better the film image, with less visible grid lines.

Focusing Distance

Focusing distance is the distance from the x-ray tube to the incident face of the grid. It is ideal to use a grid having the proper focal distance complying to the radiographic distance. If a grid having a different focal distance from the actual radiographic distance is used, part of the primary radiation which is necessary to create the film image is also absorbed along with the scatter radiation, producing a film image with insufficient exposure.

Types of Grid

The Linear Grid

In the linear grid, the strips of lead are placed parallel to each other (Fig. 5-3).

While using the linear grid, cut-off of the beam can occur as some of the primary beam may get absorbed by the lead in the peripheral region. Sometimes this can also take place in the centre of the film if the grid is not perpendicular to the central axis of the beam.

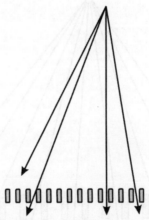

Fig. 5-3: Linear grid

Focused Grid

The disadvantage of using a linear grid can be greatly minimized by using a focused grid. In the focused grid, the lead strips are angled from the center to the edge so that the interspaces are directed at the focal spot (Fig. 5-4).

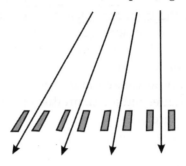

Fig. 5-4: Focused grid

Pseudofocused Grid

The extra reduction of primary radiation away from the center of the beam can be minimized by using a pseudofocused grid, in which, the height of the lead strips are progressively reduced from the center to the periphery (Fig. 5-5).

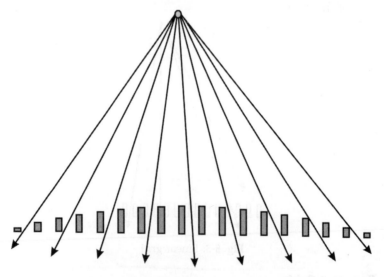

Fig. 5-5: Pseudofocused grid

Crossed Grid

Another effective way of limiting the scattered radiation further is by using a crossed grid. Here, two grids are placed on top of each other and at right angles. This minimizes the scattered radiation traversing in the same line as the primary beam.

Moving Grid (Fig. 5-6)

The use of moving grid reduces the white lead lines in the radiographic image. This is achieved by moving the grid sideways during exposure.

One of the important disadvantages of using a grid is the appearance of lead lines, which are the white lines due to the radioabsorbant material (lead) used in the grid. The use of moving grid reduces the white lead lines in the radiographic image. Moving grid is also known as Potter-Bucky grid or more commonly as Bucky grid. The moving grid is placed under the table where the x-ray film cassette is also placed. Reduction in the appearance of the lead lines is achieved by moving the grid sideways during radiation exposure. Movement of the grid facilitates the blurring out of the shadows of the lead lines. Bucky is mounted on bearings, which permit movement along rails under the x-ray table. Removal of grid lines are indicated only when superior image quality is desired. Therefore, use of moving grid has limited application in the radiography of facial region.

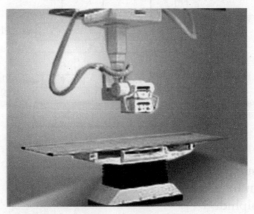

Fig. 5-6: Moving grid

INTENSIFYING SCREENS

Intensifying screens make use of the principle of fluorescence (emission of visible light). Certain inorganic salts or phosphors (e.g. magnesium oxide or titanium dioxide) have the property of absorbing x-ray photons and emitting visible light. These salts are incorporated into the intensifying screens and used along with the x-ray film. An intensifying screen and film combination makes the image receptor system 10–60 times more sensitive than when the film is used alone. Thus, the use of intensifying screens considerably reduces the radiation exposure to the patient.

The ideal requirements of a fluorescent material are:
- The material should absorb a greater amount of x-rays. Thus, it should have a high absorption coefficient
- The materials should have moderately high atomic number (Z)
- The material should emit a large amount of light of a suitable energy and color (Fig. 5-7)
- There should not be any afterglow which can adversely affect the image quality.

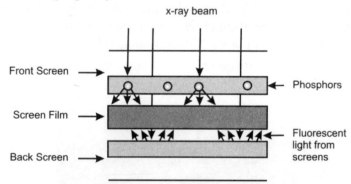

Fig. 5-7: Phosphor layer emitting visible light

The various phosphors are
- Calcium tungstate
- Zinc sulphide
- Zinc cadmium sulphide

_Barium lead sulphate
• Terbium-activated gadolinium oxysulphide (Gd_2O_2:Tb)
• Thalium-activated lanthanum oxybromide (LaOBr:Tm).

The last two phosphors in the list are rare earth materials. These phosphors are also called as 'salts', hence, the intensifying screens are also called as 'salt screens'. Calcium tungstate is the most commonly used phosphor.

Composition of Intensifying Screens (Fig. 5-8)

An intensifying screen has the following layers:
• Base
• Reflecting layer
• Phosphor layer
• Coat.

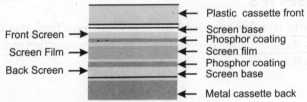

Front Screen →
Screen Film →
Back Screen →

← Plastic cassette front
← Screen base
← Phosphor coating
← Screen film
← Phosphor coating
← Screen base
← Metal cassette back

Fig. 5-8: Composition of intensifying screen

Base

Base of an intensifying screen is usually made up of polyester plastic having a thickness of 0.25 mm. The base is used for supporting the various materials that compose the screen.

Reflecting Layer

The reflecting layer is usually made of a white layer of titanium dioxide. It reflects the light emitted by the phosphor layer to the x-ray film. It lies below the phosphor layer.

Phosphor Layer

The various phosphors used are mentioned above. The rare earth intensifying screens are about four times more efficient than calcium tungstate intensifying screen. Special x-ray films sensitive to green light are required while using rare earth intensifying screens.

Coat

The protective coat is made up of plastic having a thickness of about 8 µm over the phosphor layer. It is the surface layer of the intensifying screen. This layer can be cleaned. The intensifying screen should be kept clean without any debris, spots, or scratches. Otherwise these areas will result in underexposed or light areas in the image.

The intensifying screens are used in conjunction with extraoral films. The screen-film combination is kept within light-proof cassettes. The resolving power of an intensifying screen depends on its speed. If the speed is more, the resolving power will be less and *vice versa*.

CASSETTES

Cassette is a flat box used for transporting a film and which holds the intensifying screen and film in close contact with each other (Fig. 5-9).

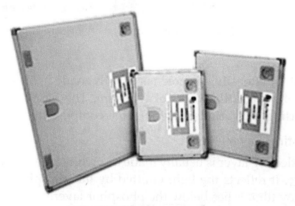

Fig. 5-9: Cassettes of different sizes

The main functions of a cassette are:
- It maintains the film in close contact with the screen during exposure
- It prevents light exposure
- It protects the intensifying screen from physical damage.

A cassette generally consists of two rectangular plates held together by hinges on a long edge. It has a front side which faces the x-ray tube and a back side which is kept away from the tube.

The ideal requirements of a cassette are:

- It should not be heavy. It should be lighter in weight for ease of handling
- It should be sufficiently strong enough to withstand daily rough handling and it should not get damaged easily
- The cassette design should be such that it can be easily handled even in the diminished light setting of a dark room.
- A cassette should have smooth outline and round corners.

Types of Cassettes

(1) *Rigid Cassettes*

A rigid cassette, as the name implies, cannot be folded or bent. It contains two metal components at the front and back to achieve the required rigidity. Rigid cassettes are predominantly used in radiography.

(2) *Curved Cassettes*

A curved cassette is used to achieve a parallel relationship between the subject and the film in certain anatomical regions with curvature. In some panoramic machines, curved cassettes are used.

(3) *Gridded Cassette*

A gridded cassette contains an incorporated grid at the front of it to minimize the scattered x-ray photons from reaching the film.

(4) *Flexible Cassette*

A flexible cassette is used for adaptation to rounded surfaces. A flexible cassette is made up of plastic. It has main application in orthopantomography.

Chapter 6

Processing of the X-ray Films

- *Introduction*
- *Latent Image*
- *Developer*
- *Developer Replenisher*
- *Fixer*
- *Fixer Replenisher*
- *Steps in Processing*
- *Darkroom*
- *Types of Processing*

So as you come and as you do depart,
Joys ebb and flow within my tender heart.

– **Charles Best**

INTRODUCTION

Processing is the collective term used for a series of operations, which bring about chemical changes in an exposed film, thus making the image visible and permanent.

When a film is exposed to radiation, there is formation of a latent image. This image becomes apparent for viewing under transillumination only if it is developed and fixed by processing. An unprocessed film is still sensitive to light and radiation. The image can be made visible and permanent only by processing (Fig. 6-1).

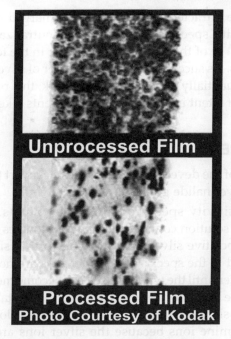

Fig. 6-1: Photomicrographic view of unprocessed and processed film

LATENT IMAGE

The film emulsion consists of positive silver and negative bromine ions that are arranged in a geometric pattern. This geometric pattern is called a crystal lattice. When a silver bromide (AgBr) grain is exposed to x-rays, some of the bromine ions present in the lattice emit electrons. These electrons travel through the crystal structure with a high mobility and get into certain locations called 'electron traps' in the crystal.

The electron trap is a region of low energy in the crystal. It is also called as sensitivity speck. As the electrons are trapped, there is a negative charge in the speck. This is one stage in the formation of a latent image.

As it has been mentioned earlier, the silver ions in the crystal have a positive charge. All the silver ions in the crystal are not held firmly and some are free to move. These ions that are freely movable are attracted to the negatively charged electrons in the sensitivity speck. Thus, there is a neutralization of the positive charge of the silver ions, resulting in the formation of silver atoms. As successively larger number of silver atoms are formed sequentially at the sensitivity speck, this results in the formation of latent image. This cycle of events takes only 10^{-11} seconds.

DEVELOPER

The action of the developing solution is to convert (reduce) the exposed silver halide grains to metallic silver.

The sensitivity speck contains silver atoms. When the developing solution contacts the silver, it donates electrons to neutralize positive silver ions allowing further silver ions to get attached to the speck. These silver ions are neutralized to metallic silver until the whole crystal has become metallic silver. The negative bromine ions which formed the crystal lattice with the positive silver ions are dispersed into the developer solution as free bromine ions because the silver ions are no longer available for keeping them.

Composition

Developing Agents

A developing agent is a substance which is capable of converting silver halide to metallic silver. The conversion of a salt or oxide to a metal is called chemical reduction.

The developing agents used are elon or metol and hydroquinone. Elon or metol brings the image rapidly. The chemical name of elon is monomethy-para-aminophenol sulfate. Hydroquinone provides high contrast to the image and does not begin development as rapidly as metol. The chemical name of hydroquinone is paradihydroxybenzene. It is very sensitive to temperature changes. It becomes highly active above 70°F and it is less active below 60°F.

In automatic processing machines, instead of elon (or metol)-hydroquinone combination, phenidone-hydroquinone combination is used. This combination results in rapid development. But there can be low contrast and film fog in the resultant radiographic image.

② *Accelerator*

The pH of the developing solution is critical for its activity. The ideal pH for developing solution is 10–11.5. Hence, the developing solution contains an alkali or accelerator. The various chemical agents used are sodium carbonate, sodium hydroxide, potassium carbonate, and potassium hydroxide. Potassium salts are more soluble than sodium salts.

③ *Restrainer or Retarder*

The function of the restrainer is to prevent the action of developer on the unexposed silver halide grains and thus to prevent film fog. In the absence of the restrainer, the developer will be very active and reduces even the unexposed grains. This action is suppressed by increasing the barrier of negatively charged bromine ions existing around the silver bromide crystals. The restrainer used is potassium bromide. In phenidone-hydroquinone system, in addition to potassium bromide, benzotriazole is also used.

④ *Preservative*

A preservative is added to prevent the oxidation of the developing solution. Sodium sulphite and potassium sulphite are used as preservatives. The action of the sulphite preservative is to form sulphonates with the early oxidation products.

⑤ *Solvent*

Water, which is cheap and universally available is used as the solvent.

In addition to the basic components, the developing solution also contains water softeners, wetting agents, and bactericidal substances.

DEVELOPER REPLENISHER

The replenisher is added every day to the processing solution to top off so as to maintain its chemical activity. The replenisher generally has the same composition as the developing solution. But, the developer-replenisher is more alkaline and does not contain restraining bromide.

FIXER

When a film is taken out from the developer, the exposed and developed silver halide crystals have become black metallic silver and an image has already formed. The unexposed silver halide crystals are not developed. As those unexposed crystals are still light-sensitive, they have to be removed. Therefore, the action of the fixing solution is to remove the unexposed silver halide crystals. The fixing solution also hardens the emulsion which was softened by the developing solution.

Composition

① The Fixing Agent

The action of the fixing agent is to react with silver halide to form a soluble compound without any appreciable effect on the metallic silver image which has already been formed. Sodium thiosulphate or (hypo) is used as the fixing agent.

In some liquid concentrates, ammonium thiosulphate is used as a fixing agent.

② Acidifier

The action of the acidifier is to neutralize any alkali of the developing solution which is still adherent to the film. The acidifier also limits the action of any alkaline developer which may be left in the film. The acidifier commonly used is a weak acid such as acetic acid. The acidifier usually creates a pH range of 4.0-5.0.

③ Hardener

The emulsion layer of the film absorbs considerable moisture and swells during processing. A swollen emulsion facilitates the action of the various ingredients of the developing solution. The function of the hardener is to harden the emulsion. Various hardeners used are chrome potassium alum, potassium alum, and aluminium chloride.

Solvent

In fixing solution also, the solvent used is water.

Other addition in a fixing solution is boric acid which functions as an antisludging agent.

FIXER REPLENISHER

The fixing solution constantly gets diluted as water from the rinse is carried in and fixer is carried out. There is also an accumulation of soluble silver complexes (argentothio-sulphates) and soluble halides. As a result of these changes, the time taken for fixing becomes longer. The fixer-replenisher contains a fixing agent (ammonium thiosulphate), acetic acid, a hardener such as aluminium chloride, and sodium sulphite as a preservative.

STEPS IN PROCESSING

Processing consists of the following steps:
- Immersion of an exposed film in the developing solution
- Rinsing in water
- Immersion in the fixing solution
- Film washing in running water
- Drying and mounting for viewing.

Immersion in Developing Solution

The action of the developing solution has already been discussed. An exposed film is immersed in the developing solution until the image emerges. Depending on the exposure time, mA, kVp, and the concentration of the developing solution, the time taken for development ranges from a few seconds to few minutes.

Rinsing in Water

Rinsing in water is done after the film is developed. The film should be rinsed in water for 15–20 seconds before placing in the fixer. It slows down the development process and removes any alkali of the developing solution before placing in acidic fixer.

Immersion in the Fixing Solution

As it has already been discussed, the action of the fixing solution is to remove the unexposed silver halide crystals and harden the emulsion. It takes about 20 minutes for the fixing action to complete. Too long fixing time can cause film fog and loss of proper contrast.

Film Washing

After fixing, the film should be washed thoroughly for sufficient length of time in running water. If the silver compounds are not removed, there can be stains on the film. Discoloration of the image can also result due to the presence of thiosulphate and its products.

Drying and Mounting for Viewing

The last step in the processing is film drying and mounting for viewing. The film should be kept in a dust-free area for drying. The films may be hung by using clips or holders. Commercially, driers are available for drying the film. It is a large chamber in which there is facility for hanging the wet film. A coil within the chamber is electrically heated to generate heat. A fan inside the chamber helps in the circulation of hot air. Drying a film is very important as sometimes the water marks can result in artefacts. The processed films should be properly identified, mounted, and then viewed under transillumination.

DARKROOM

Manual processing is done in a darkroom with safelight illumination. Safelight refers to the light with a particular wavelength which does not significantly affect the radiographic film. The illuminator is situated near the site of handling the wet film. Exposure of film for longer than normal time in the safelighting conditions can adversely affect the image. Safelighting can be provided by red, brown, or olive-green lighting. Safe illumination is usually provided by an ordinary bulb of not more than 25 watts with a colored filter placed in front of the bulb to achieve the required hue. Safelighting can either be direct or indirect.

In direct safelighting, the lamp has a circular filter 14 cm (5.5 inches) in diameter and fixed either to the ceiling or to the wall above the working bench. The safelight should be kept at least 4 feet above the place where the film is handled.

Indirect safelighting is provided by a safelight which is directed to the ceiling from where it is reflected back to the room.

TYPES OF PROCESSING

There are basically two types of processing methods. They are:
1. Manual processing
   - Visual method
   - Time-temperature method.
2. Automatic processing.

Manual Processing

Visual Method

The visual method of manual processing is carried out in a darkroom with safelighting conditions. In this method, an exposed x-ray film is immersed in the developing solution and periodically viewed under the safelight for the emergence of a clear image. When the image appears the film is washed and immersed in the fixing solution. Figure 6-2 shows the placement of processing tanks.

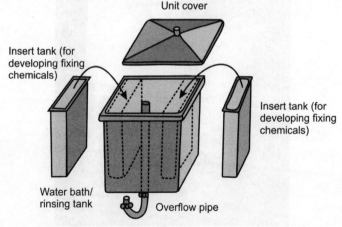

Fig. 6-2: Placement of processing tanks

Time-temperature Method

Time-temperature method is a type of manual processing method in which effective standardization may be achieved without any automatic aids. This is a simple technique of immersing the film in the developer kept at a constant temperature for a fixed duration of time. The time-temperature chart is given in Table 6-1.

Though the manual processing has a clear advantage that the action of development is under the direct control of the operator, there is a necessity to handle wet film and the requirement of a darkroom. Manual processing is also time consuming.

Table 6-1: Time-temperature chart

Temperature	Development time
65°F	6 minutes
68°F	5 minutes
70°F	4.5 minutes
72°F	4 minutes
76°F	3 minutes
80°F	2.5 minutes

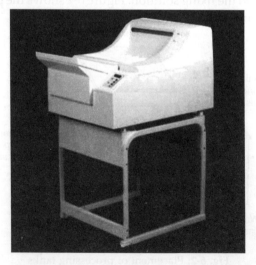

Fig. 6-3: An automatic film processor

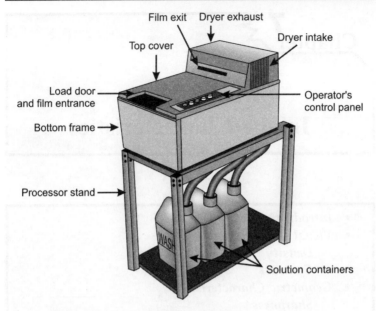

Fig. 6-4: Diagrammatic representation of automatic
x-ray film processor

Automatic Processing

In automatic processing machines (Fig. 6-3), the exposed film
is fed at one end of the processor and it passes successively
through the developer, fixer, water, and drier. In automatic
processing, the step of rinsing in water after developing is
avoided. As the roller system has a squeezing action, the
developing solution absorbed by the gelatin of the emulsion
will be less as it is transported from the developer to the fixer.

The automatic processing machines make use of belt-driven
roller system for the transport of film. The temperature of the
processing solution is also maintained. The film comes out
through the other end of the processor, processed, dry, and
ready for viewing (Fig. 6-4).

Chapter 7

Dental X-ray Image Characteristics

- *Introduction*
- *Visual Characteristics*
    Density
    Contrast
- *Geometric Characteristics*
    Sharpness
    Magnification
    Distortion
    Image Resolution
- *Factors Influencing Diagnostic Quality of a Radiograph*

Think, if thou on beauty leanest,
Think how pitiful that stay,
Did not virtue give the meanest
Charms superior to decay

– William Wordsworth

INTRODUCTION

The characteristics of a radiographic image are the visual characteristics such as density and contrast and geometric characteristics such as sharpness, magnification, and distortion. An ideal radiograph should have these characteristics in the optimal level. Apart from these characteristics, for proper radiographic diagnosis, the intraoral periapical radiograph should represent the area radiographed and it should be devoid of any technical errors.

A dental radiograph appears as black (radiolucent) and white (radiopaque) image and also includes varying degrees of gray shade. A radiolucent image is produced due to the lack of density of the object, permitting passage of x-ray beam without any attenuation. A radiopaque image is produced by dense structures that absorb and resist the passage of x-ray beam. For example, the mineralized structures such as enamel, dentin, and bone cast radiopaque shadow.

An ideal radiograph is one that provides a great deal of required information, with the images exhibiting proper density and contrast, and having sharp outlines; same shape; and same size.

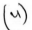 VISUAL CHARACTERISTICS

Density

Density refers to overall darkening of a radiograph. Density depends on the degree of silver blackening in the exposed and processed radiograph. If the density is too high, the images appear dark with poor diagnostic quality. Conversely, if the density is less, the contrast will be improper.

Density depends on milliamperage (mA), kilovoltage peak (kVp), and exposure time. Density also depends on the subject thickness and development conditions.

Contrast

Contrast refers to the difference in the contrasting radio-densities or it is the difference in the degrees of blackness between adjacent areas in a dental radiograph. In a radiograph with ideal contrast, the dark and light areas should be strikingly different.

Film contrast is the characteristics of a film influencing the radiographic contrast. This is dependent on the qualities of the film and film processing.

Subject contrast is the characteristics of the object influencing the radiographic contrast. These factors are the thickness, density, and composition of the subject.

The radiographic contrast depends on kVp. If kVp is increased, the contrast becomes less and *vice versa*. It also depends on mA, exposure time, and processing conditions.

A radiograph that exhibits only two densities (areas of black and white) has a 'short-scale contrast', whereas, a radiograph that exhibits many densities (many shades of gray) has a 'long-contrast scale'. Scales of contrast can be measured by using a device called stepwedge. It consists of aluminium steps in 2-mm increments. When a stepwedge is placed on top of a film and exposed to x-rays, each step absorbs varying amounts of x-rays, resulting in different film densities appearing in the radiograph.

GEOMETRIC CHARACTERISTICS

Sharpness

Sharpness of the radiographic image refers to how well a boundary between two contrasting radiodensities is delineated. Sharpness depends on focal spot size, film composition, and any movement of the subject or film during exposure. A fuzzy, unclear area surrounding a radiographic image is termed 'penumbra' (Latin, pene meaning almost and umbra meaning shadow). A penumbra is defined as the sharpness or blurring of the periphery of a radiographic image.

Magnification

Magnification is the term given for a radiographic image which appears larger than the actual size of the object which was radiographed. To a greater extent, the magnification occurs due to the divergent nature of the x-ray beam. The other factors influencing magnification are decrease in target to object distance and increase in object to film distance as well as large effective focal spot.

Distortion

Distortion refers to a variation in the size or shape of the object being radiographed. The various factors contributing to the distortion of the image are improper object-film alignment (ideally the object and film must be parallel to each other) or improper x-ray beam angulation (ideally the central x-ray beam should be perpendicular to the object and the film).

Image Resolution

Image resolution is a measure of visualization of relatively small objects that are close together as separate objects. Sharpness and resolution are determined by the same geometric variables.

FACTORS INFLUENCING DIAGNOSTIC QUALITY OF A RADIOGRAPH

Most of the influencing factors required for the optimum diagnostic quality of a radiograph have already been discussed in different sections in this book. Hence these factors are only enumerated here. The reader is requested to refer the appropriate sections for further information.

- Milliamperage (mA)
- Kilovoltage peak (kVp)
- Exposure time
- Density of the object
- Speed of the film
- Collimation
- Source to object distance
- Object to film distance
- Inverse square law
- Ideal technique and processing conditions
- Good quality of x-ray film
- Use of small effective focal spot.

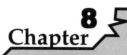

Chapter 8

Causes of Faulty Radiographs

- *Introduction*
- *Faulty Radiographs Resulting from Faulty Radiographic Techniques*
- *Faulty Radiographs Resulting from Faulty Processing Techniques*

One said: Thy life is thine to make or mar,
To flicker feebly, or to soar, a star;
It lies with thee - the choice is thine, is thine,
To hit the ties or drive thy autocar.

– Robert WS

INTRODUCTION

Faulty radiographs are nondiagnostic radiographs in the sense that these radiographs are of no diagnostic value as they do not provide adequate detail and required information. A diagnostic radiograph is one that provides a great deal of information; the images have proper density and contrast, have sharp outlines, and the structures are of the same size and shape as that of the object radiographed.

The problems encountered in radiographic images are due to faulty technique of radiography or faulty technique of processing. Accordingly, there can be partial or total absence of images, films are light, dark, yellow-brown and fogged; or there are scratched emulsion or fingerprints.

This chapter deals with various faulty radiographs and their causes. Various methods for avoiding these faults are self-explanatory.

FAULTY RADIOGRAPHS RESULTING FROM FAULTY RADIOGRAPHIC TECHNIQUES

Foreshortening of the Image

Foreshortening or shortening refers to images of the teeth and other structures that appear too short. In an ideal radiograph, the structures imaged should have the same size and shape. Foreshortening results from excessive vertical angulation of the x-ray tube during radiography. It is imperative that appropriate vertical angulations must be used while taking radiographs. Foreshortening of the image can adversely affect the treatment planning as well as the outcome of the treatment.

Elongation of the Image

Elongation refers to images of the teeth and associated structures that appear too long than real.

Elongation of image results from decreased vertical angulation. Therefore, it is important that appropriate vertical angulations must be used while taking intraoral periapical radiographs.

Elongation of a Few Teeth

Elongation of a few teeth refers to a few teeth appearing longer than normal, whereas other teeth are of normal size.

Elongation of a few teeth results from excessive bending of the film in an attempt to place in the patient's mouth. In the bent portion of the film the image appears elongated. In an attempt to cause less discomfort to the patient, the film should not be bent excessively. Only a gentle bend must be given to the film just for conforming to the anatomical contour of the intraoral structures such as the palate and the floor of the mouth. There is also a chance for bending of the film when canine-premolar areas are radiographed.

Overlapping of Proximal Surfaces

Overlapping of proximal surfaces results from improper horizontal angulation. Overlapping of proximal surfaces makes the radiographs of less diagnostic value, especially in the detection of proximal caries.

Slanting of Occlusal Plane or Incisal Plane

In an ideal radiograph, the occlusal plane or incisal plane should be parallel to the margin of the film.

Slanting of occlusal plane results from improper placement of the film in the patient's mouth.

Image of Coronal Portion of the Teeth not Seen Completely

The image of coronal portion of the teeth is cut off due to improper placement of the film in the patient's mouth. Sufficient area of the film should be visible between the incisal or occlusal plane and the margin of the film. This is to ensure that the image of the coronal portion of the teeth is seen fully.

Image of the Apical Region not Seen

In some radiographs, the periapical region of the required tooth may not be visualized fully. In such situations, radiographic diagnosis is not possible.

Sufficient area of the periapical region should be visible in a radiograph for better diagnostic use. This concept is readily apparent in the evaluation of any pathology involving the periapical region. The image in the periapical region is cut off due to improper placement of the film in the patient's mouth.

Blurred or Distorted Image

Blurred or distorted image refers to an image which appears hazy and without any sharpness.

Blurred or distorted image is due to either the movement of the patient, the film placed in the patient's mouth, or the x-ray tube during exposure.

Cone-cut Appearance

Cone-cut appearance refers to a clear, unexposed area in a dental radiograph. In the rest of the area of the film, image is seen.

This fault results from the x-ray beam not centered over the film, or in other words, if the central x-ray is not perpendicular to the center of the film (Fig. 8-1).

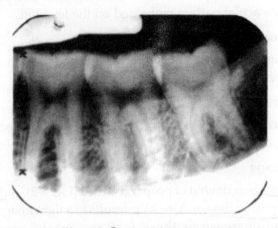

Fig. 8-1: Cone-cut appearance

Phalangioma

The term phalangioma was used by Dr David F Mitchell of the Indiana University School of Dentistry. It refers to the image of phalanx (*plural*—phalanges) appearing in the film.

Phalangioma occurs when the patient holds the film in the mouth in an incorrect way leading to the appearance of the image of the fingers in the radiograph. It must be remembered that finger-holding method of intraoral radiography is not advised as per the radiation protection protocols.

Double Exposure or Double Image

Double exposure or double image refers to appearance of two separate images in the radiograph.

Double exposure or double image appears due to repeated exposure of an already exposed film.

Reversed Film

Reversed film refers to a film exposed from the opposite side.

If the film is placed in the mouth reversed and then exposed, the x-ray beam gets attenuated by the lead foil backing in the film packet. It decreases the amount of x-ray beam exposing the film. This results in light images with herringbone or tyre-track or car-tyre appearance in the radiograph. This pattern is due to the actual pattern embossed on the lead foil.

Film Creasing

Film creasing can result either in cracking of emulsion or a thin radiolucent line appears in the radiograph.

Crimp-marks

Crimp-marks or nail-like curved dark lines result from sharp bending of the film.

Light Image

A light image is devoid of proper contrast (Fig. 8-2). A decrease in the exposure time, mA, or kVp results in a light image. Apart from the decrease in these factors, certain processing errors can also result in light image. These factors are discussed below.

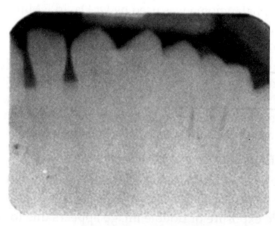

Fig. 8-2: Light radiograph

Dark Image

A dark image results from excessive exposure time, mA, or kVp (Fig. 8-3). Apart from these factors, certain processing parameters can also result in a dark image. These factors are also discussed below.

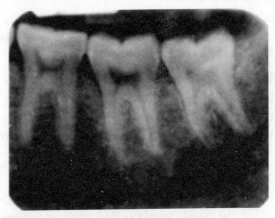

Fig. 8-3: Dark radiograph

FAULTY RADIOGRAPHS RESULTING FROM FAULTY PROCESSING TECHNIQUES

Light Image

Apart from less exposure time, mA, and kVp, a light image can also result from inadequate development time, inaccurate timer, low developer temperature, and depleted or contaminated developing solution.

Dark Image

A dark image is the result of excessive development time, inaccurate timer, higher developer temperature, and concentrated developer solution.

Cracked or Reticulated Image

Cracked or reticulated image results when the film is subjected to a sudden temperature change between the developer and the water bath.

Dark Spots on the Film

Dark spots (developer spots) on the film occur due to droplets of developing solution coming in contact with an exposed film before it is developed.

White Spots on the Film

White spots (fixer spots) on the film results from droplets of fixing solution coming in contact with an exposed film before it is developed.

Blank Film

Blank film refers to total absence of image. The film appears translucent as the entire emulsion is washed off. This results from immersing the exposed film in the fixing solution before it is immersed in the developing solution.

White Area on the Film

When two films come in contact with each other during development, the overlapped portion appears whiter.

Dark Areas on the Film

Dark areas appear on film when overlap has occurred in the fixer.

Straight White Border

If the level of the developing solution is too low, the film will not be fully immersed in the developer, resulting in a straight white border representing the undeveloped portion of the film.

Straight Black Border

If the level of the fixer is too low, in the unfixed portion of the film, straight black border appears.

White Marks on the Film

When air bubbles are trapped on the film surface, the processing solution does not come in contact with the film. This results in white marks on the film.

Nail Marks

Nail mark artefacts are crescent-shaped when the emulsion is damaged by the fingernail due to rough handling of the film.

Thin Black Branching Lines or Tree-like Appearance

This appearance results from static electricity exposing the film due to the following reasons:
- Opening of the film packet too quickly
- Humid conditions
- Rubbing of the film with the intensifying screen.

Fingermarks

Fingermarks on the film result from handling the film with wet finger.

Scratched Emulsion

When the film comes in contact with sharp objects, the emulsion in that area is removed, causing scratched emulsion as in these areas the emulsion has peeled off.

Light Exposure

Due to light exposure, the exposed portion of the film appears black.

Fogged Film

Fogged film refers to a film which appears gray without image detail and contrast. This fault results from improper safelighting conditions, light leakage, improper storage conditions of the film, expired or outdated film, contaminated processing solution, or high temperature of the developer.

Chapter

Intraoral Radiographic Techniques and Indications for Intraoral Radiographs

THE *world's an inn; and I her guest,*
I eat; I drink; I take my rest.
My hostess, nature, does deny me
Nothing, wherewith she can supply me;
Where, having stayed a while, I pay
Her lavish bills, and go my way.

– Francis Quarles

INTRODUCTION

Basically there are two techniques for taking intraoral radiographs. These techniques are:
1. Paralleling technique and
2. Bisecting angle technique.

PARALLELING TECHNIQUE (FIG. 9-1)

Paralleling technique is also called as the extension cone paralleling technique (XCP), right angle technique, and long-cone technique.

As the name implies, this technique is based on the concept of parallelism. In this technique, the film is placed in the mouth parallel to the long axis of the tooth and the central x-ray beam is directed perpendicular to or at a right angle to the long axis of the tooth and the film.

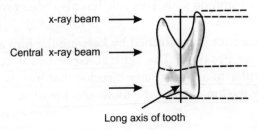

Fig. 9-1: Diagrammatic representation of paralleling technique

This technique employs special holders to achieve this parallelism. These holders are Rinn XCP Instruments (X-extended, C-cone, and P-paralleling), and precision film holders.

This technique is performed by keeping the film far away from the teeth surface to achieve parallelism. As position indicating devices (PID) are used, there is no specific head position or vertical angulation for orienting the x-ray tube. This technique employs long lead-lined cones having a length of 12–16 inches. The film is kept parallel to the long axis of the tooth and, the central x-ray beam must be directed perpendicular to the long axis of the tooth and the film. The horizontal angulation is such that the central x-ray beam must be directed through the contact area between the teeth, and the x-ray tube conforms to the PID. The PIDs help in directing the central x-ray beam to the center of the film.

An advantage of this technique is that errors due to improper placement of the film are minimized and the magnification of the image is negligible or not there at all.

The paralleling technique cannot be performed in edentulous patients and in patients with shallow floor of the mouth and shallow palate.

BISECTING ANGLE TECHNIQUE (Fig. 9-2)

Bisecting angle technique is also called as bisecting technique, bisection-of-the-angle technique, and short-cone technique. This technique is based on Cieszynski's rule of isometry which states that two triangles are equal if they have two equal angles and have a common side. This rule has also been proposed by Weston A. Price.

This technique is performed by keeping the film as close to the teeth as possible. The central x-ray beam is directed perpendicular to an imaginary bisector that bisects the angle formed by the long axis of the tooth and the film.

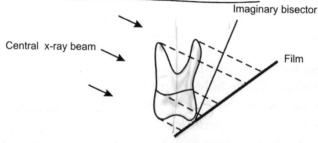

Fig. 9-2: Diagrammatic representation of bisecting angle technique

The imaginary bisector creates two equal angles and provides a common side for the two imaginary equal triangles. The two imaginary triangles are right angles and are congruent. The hypotenuse of the imaginary triangle is represented by the long axis of the tooth and the other hypotenuse is represented by the vertical plane of the film.

While performing this technique, specific head alignment and specific vertical angulations are necessary. The central x-ray beam should be perpendicular to the imaginary bisector bisecting the angle formed by the long axis of the tooth and the film. The horizontal angulation is adjusted in such a way that the central x-ray beam is centered through the contact area between the teeth.

Specialized holders are not necessary for performing this technique. This technique can be performed by finger-holding

A.R. BOOK POINT

CASH MEMO   Cell : 8121787892

All kinds of Books Available - Old & New Books on Rental Basis

S.No. 20, Backside Clock Tower, C.B.I. Office,
M.C.H. Commercial Complex, Sultan Bazar, Koti, Hyderabad.

679

No. ....

Date...3/6/24.....

Mr./ Mrs. / Ms. .... Dental Books

S. NO.	PARTICULARS	RATE	AMOUNT Rs. Ps.
①	Surgery Chitra 9th	9th	610
②	Radiogy 3rd ed	9th	450

Thank You   Visit Again !   **TOTAL**   1080

For A.R. BOOK POI...

M.C.H. Comercial Complex, Sultan Bazar, Koti, Hyderabad.

679

No. ....   Date 31.01.20..

Mr/ Mrs/ Ms. .... Priya Books

S. No.	PARTICULARS	RATE	AMOUNT Rs. P.
(1)	Surgical CANUKA 937		670
	1853		
(2)	Radiology Jha 493		450
	Next Again Thank You	TOTAL	1120

A.R.
For A.R. BOOK POINT

method. However, for radiation protection, it is safe to use holders.

The various vertical angulations to be followed while performing this technique are given in Table 9-1.

Table 9-1: Different vertical angulations

Teeth	Maxillary vertical angulation in degrees	Mandibular vertical angulation in degrees
Incisors	+50	−20
Canine	+45	−15
Premolar	+30	−10
Molar	+25	−5 (for first and second molars)
		0 (for third molars)

*Vertical angulation for bitewing radiographs +5.

INDICATIONS FOR INTRAORAL PERIAPICAL RADIOGRAPH

The indications for intraoral periapical (IOPA) radiographs are enumerated below:
- To visualize periapical region
- In the diagnosis of periapical pathology
- To study crown and root length
- To determine root morphology
- To study the integrity of the lamina dura
- Selection of cases for endodontic treatment
- During and after endodontic treatment
- In the evaluation of fracture of the teeth
- As part of routine radiographic examination
- To evaluate root apex formation
- To study eruption pattern and stage of eruption
- To identify impacted teeth, supernumerary teeth, and root stumps
- Presurgical evaluation
- Postsurgical evaluation of the socket
- To evaluate site for implant placement
- During the fabrication of crown and bridge, to evaluate the status or condition of adjacent teeth

- In the evaluation of a reimplanted tooth
- Follow-up evaluation after traumatic injury
- Follow-up evaluation after endodontic treatment or implant placement.

INDICATIONS FOR BITEWING RADIOGRAPH

- In the diagnosis of interproximal caries
- To study the height of the pulp chamber
- In the diagnosis of secondary caries
- To study the height of the alveolar bone or assessment of bone loss
- In the diagnosis of pulp stone
- To study occlusion of the teeth.

OCCLUSAL PROJECTION

The occlusal radiograph is taken separately for the maxilla and the mandible. Occlusal projection is an intraoral radiographic technique. Individual films are available in flexible film packets.

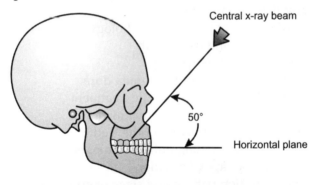

Fig. 9-3: Maxillary occlusal projection

Maxillary Occlusal Projection (Fig. 9-3)

There are three types of maxillary occlusal projection. They are:
1. Maxillary topographic occlusal projection
2. Maxillary lateral occlusal projection
3. Right-angle technique.

In anterior topographic projection, the film packet is placed in the patient's mouth with the front of the film packet facing the palate and the longer dimension of the film across the mouth. The patient is asked to gently bite on the film packet. The patient's head is positioned in such a way that the horizontal plane of the film is parallel to the floor. The central x-ray beam is directed at a vertical angulation of +50 to +60 and exiting through the root of the nose. Figure 9-4 shows a maxillary occlusal radiograph.

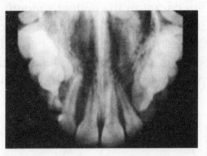

Fig. 9-4: Maxillary occlusal radiograph

In the maxillary lateral occlusal projection, the film after placing in the mouth is shifted to the side of interest or the area to be radiographed (Fig. 9-5). The central x-ray beam is directed perpendicular to the center of the film.

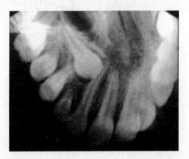

Fig. 9-5: Maxillary lateral occlusal projection

In the right-angle occlusal view of the maxilla, the film is placed in the same position in the patient's mouth as in the case of first projection. The central x-ray beam is directed perpendicular to the center of the film packet from above the head of the patient at about the hairline. The vertical angulation is +90 degrees. As the focal spot to film distance is more, this projection requires an increase in the exposure time.

Mandibular Occlusal Projection (Fig. 9-6)

Mandibular occlusal projection helps in the visualization of the entire mandibular arch. This technique is performed by keeping the film packet in the patient's mouth in such a way that the front of the film faces the mandibular occlusal surface. The patient is asked to extend the neck backwards. The x-ray tube is kept below the chin region and the central x-ray beam should be perpendicular to the floor of the mouth and the center of the film.

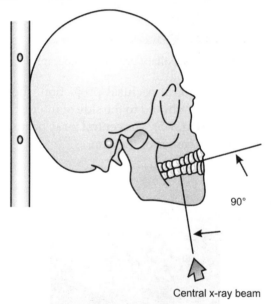

Central x-ray beam

Fig. 9-6: Mandibular occlusal projection

Indications of Occlusal Radiographs

- To study maxillary and mandibular arches
- To determine buccolingual position of impacted teeth as part of localization

- To identify expansion of the cortical plate in case of any pathology such as cysts
- To study expansion of palatal arch during orthodontic jaw expansion procedure
- Evaluation of fracture of the jaws with displacement
- Localization of objects in the maxillary sinus
- To locate stones in the duct of the submandibular gland
- To evaluate the boundaries of the maxillary sinus
- To examine cleft palate
- To measure the changes in the size and shape of the maxilla and the mandible.

Chapter 10

Normal Anatomic Landmarks

- *Introduction*
- *Anatomic Landmarks Common to the Maxilla and the Mandible*
- *Anatomic Landmarks in the Maxilla*
- *Anatomic Landmarks in the Mandible*

WHEN I have fears that I may cease to be
Before my pen has glean'd my teeming brain,
Before high piled books, in charact'ry,
Hold like rich garners the full-ripen'd grain;

– John Keats

INTRODUCTION

Various anatomic landmarks visualized in the intraoral periapical radiographs may be grouped broadly as those common to the maxilla and the mandible, those landmarks of the maxilla, and those landmarks of the mandible.

Various anatomic structures common to both the maxilla and the mandible are the teeth and the supporting structures.

ANATOMIC LANDMARKS COMMON TO THE MAXILLA AND THE MANDIBLE

Enamel

The enamel is the highly mineralized structure of the human body. It is about 92% mineralized. It is the outermost radiopaque layer of the coronal part of the teeth and radiographically it appears as an 'enamel cap'.

Dentin

The dentin is present below the enamel and surrounds the pulp cavity. It constitutes the greater bulk of the tooth structure. It is about 70% mineralized. Its radiodensity is less than that of the enamel.

Cementum

The cementum covers the root surface. It is about 65% mineralized, which is almost similar to that of dentin. Hence, radiographically it may not be possible to differentiate between the two.

Pulp Cavity

The pulp cavity is composed of pulp chamber and root canals. It is the soft tissue element of the tooth, containing blood vessels, nerves, and lymphatics. It gives a radiolucent image in the radiograph. The pulp chamber is larger in children and becomes smaller in adults due to the formation of secondary dentin.

Supporting Structures of the Teeth

The alveolar bone or the alveolar process supports the teeth in their sockets. It is composed of dense cortical bone and thin cancellous bone.

The lamina dura is the term given for a thin radiopaque line surrounding the roots of the teeth. It is the alveolar bone proper which forms the socket of the teeth. The loss of integrity of the lamina dura correlates with periapical pathology.

The alveolar crest is the coronal portion of the alveolar bone, found between the teeth. Radiographically it is located 1.5–2.0 mm below the cementoenamel junction as a dense cortical bone continuous with the lamina dura. The alveolar crest in the anterior region appears pointed and in the posterior region appears flat.

The periodontal ligament space is the space between the roots of the teeth and the lamina dura. It contains connective tissue fibers, blood vessels, and lymphatics. Radiographically it appears as a thin radiolucent line around the roots of a tooth.

Cortical Bone

The term cortical originates from the Latin word *'cortex'*, meaning outer layer. It is also called as the compact bone. It gives a radiopaque shadow in the radiograph.

Cancellous Bone

The term *'cancellous'* in Latin means 'arranged like a lattice'. It is the soft spongy bone present between the layers of dense cortical bone. It contains numerous bony trabeculae forming lattice-like network of intercommunicating spaces which are filled with bone marrow. The trabeculae are mineralized, whereas the marrow spaces permit the passage of x-ray beam.

The trabeculae in the anterior region of the maxilla are thin, numerous, and forming very fine, granular, and dense pattern. In the posterior region of the maxilla the trabecular pattern is essentially similar, but with relatively larger marrow spaces.

The trabeculae are thicker in the mandibular anterior region. It gives a coarser pattern in the radiograph. The trabeculae are few and arranged in a horizontal pattern. The marrow spaces are larger. In the posterior region of the mandible, the trabeculae and marrow spaces are larger. The trabeculae are arranged in a horizontal pattern. In some areas the trabeculae may be virtually absent, whereas in some regions they may be highly irregular in pattern.

ANATOMIC LANDMARKS IN THE MAXILLA

Incisive Foramen

The incisive foramen is also called as the nasopalatine foramen. It is a small ovoid or round radiolucent area located between the roots of the maxillary central incisors. It is located in the anterior portion of the hard palate directly posterior to the maxillary central incisors.

Superior Foramina of the Incisive Canal

The superior foramina of the incisive canal are two openings located on the floor of the nasal cavity. These two small canals join together to form the incisive canal. Nasopalatine nerves and vessels pass through these canals to exit at the incisive foramen. Rarely superior foramina of the nasopalatine canal may be visualized as two small round radiolucencies located superior to the apices of the maxillary central incisors.

Median Palatal Suture

The median palatal suture is also called as the midpalatine suture. It is the site of fusion of the palatine processes of the maxilla. It extends from the alveolar crest between the maxillary central incisors to the posterior hard palate. Radiographically it appears as a thin radiolucent line between the roots of the maxillary central incisors.

Lateral Fossa

The lateral fossa is also called as the canine fossa. It is a depression located just inferior and medial to the infraorbital foramen between the canine and the lateral incisor. Radiographically it appears as a radiolucent area between the maxillary canine and the lateral incisor. In some cases it may be absent.

Nasal Fossa

The nasal fossa is a pear-shaped cavity present superior to the oral cavity. It is visualized in the maxillary anterior radiograph as two separate radiolucent areas on either side of the nasal septum and above the maxillary incisors.

Nasal Septum

The nasal septum is a vertically placed wall that divides the nasal cavity into the right and the left nasal fossae. The nasal septum is formed by the vomer and a portion of the ethmoid bone and cartilaginous tissue. The nasal septum is seen as a vertical radiopaque partition dividing the nasal cavity.

Anterior Nasal Spine

The anterior nasal spine is a sharp projection of the maxilla located at the anterior and inferior portion of the nasal cavity. In a maxillary anterior radiograph it appears as a 'V'-shaped radiopaque structure at the junction of the nasal septum and the floor of the nasal cavity.

Inferior Nasal Conchae

The *'concha'* in Latin means shell-shaped or scroll-shaped. The inferior nasal conchae or the inferior nasal turbinates are thin curved plate of bone extending from the lateral portion of the nasal cavity. In a maxillary anterior periapical radiograph it appears as a diffuse radiopaque mass within the nasal cavity.

Maxillary Sinus (Fig. 10-1)

Maxillary sinus is a paired compartment present within the maxilla. The maxillary sinus is present above the maxillary molar and premolar teeth and rarely extending anteriorly to the canine region. Posteriorly it can extend to the maxillary tuberosity region. The maxillary sinus may also extend into the interdental bone, furcation areas of the maxillary molars, or extraction socket. In the radiograph it appears as a radiolucent area above the apices of the premolars and molars. The floor of the maxillary sinus is composed of dense cortical bone.

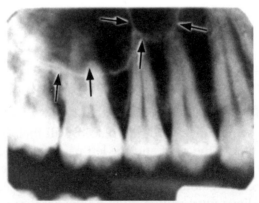

Fig. 10-1: Maxillary sinus

Sometimes bony compartments or septae may be seen within the maxillary sinus. In radiographs, the septae appear as radiopaque lines dividing the sinus into compartments and imparting a multilocular appearance.

In some radiographs there may be narrow radiolucent bands with radiopaque border that represent nutrient canals of the maxillary sinus.

Inverted 'Y' Configuration

The inverted 'Y'-shaped configuration is formed by the merging of the anterior border of maxillary sinus and the lateral wall of the nasal fossa. This configuration is seen in the canine or the premolar region.

Maxillary Tuberosity

The maxillary tuberosity is a round prominence that extends posteriorly beyond the third molar region. In the periapical radiographs of the maxillary posterior region it appears as a radiopaque bulge distal to the third molar region.

Hamular Process

The hamular process is also known as the hamulus. It is a projection of bone extending down from the medial pterygoid plate of the sphenoid bone. It is located posterior to the maxillary tuberosity. Radiographically it appears as a radiopaque hook-like projection distal to the maxillary tuberosity.

Medial and Lateral Pterygoid Plates

The medial and the lateral pterygoid plates are located posterior to the maxillary tuberosity. The shape and size of the pterygoid plates may vary. In some radiographs they may not be visualized at all. They appear as a single homogeneous shadow without any trabeculae.

Zygomatic Process of the Maxilla

The bony projection, the zygomatic process of the maxilla, articulates with the malar bone. It is composed of dense cortical bone. In a maxillary periapical radiograph it appears as a

'U'-shaped radiopaque band located above the maxillary first molar region (Fig. 10-2).

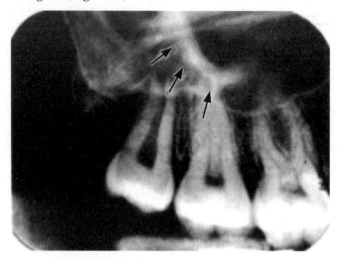

Fig. 10-2: Zygomatic process of maxilla

Zygomatic (Malar) Bone

In the periapical radiograph of the maxillary posterior region, the lower part of the zygomatic bone may be seen extending posteriorly from the border of the zygomatic process of the maxilla. It appears as a uniform gray radiopacity over the apical region of the molars.

ANATOMIC LANDMARKS IN THE MANDIBLE

Genial Tubercles

The genial tubercles are tiny projections from the lingual aspect of the mandible, serving as attachment sites for the genioglossus and the geniohyoid muscles. In a mandibular intraoral periapical radiograph they appear as tiny circular radiopacity below the apical region of the central incisors.

Lingual Foramen

The lingual foramen is situated near the midline on the internal surface of the mandible and is surrounded by the genial tubercle. Radiographically it appears as a small radiolucent foramen below the apical region of the central incisors.

Nutrient Canals

The nutrient canals are tubular passageways through bone, containing nerves and blood vessels supplying the teeth. The nutrient canals are more apparent in the mandibular anterior region due to the relatively thin bone. In the periapical radiograph these nutrient canals appear as vertical radiolucent lines, in edentulous patients the nutrient canals are more prominent. The nutrient canals may be mistaken for fracture lines.

Mental Ridge

The mental ridge is a linear, thick bony prominence in the anterior portion of the mandible. It extends from the premolar region to the midline and is directed upwards. In the periapical radiographs, it appears as an inverted 'V'-shaped thick radiopaque band.

Mental Fossa

The mental fossa is a depressed area on the external surface of the mandibular anterior region above the mental ridge. In the mandibular periapical radiograph it appears as a radiolucent area above the mental ridge.

Mental Foramen

The mental foramen is located on the outer surface of the mandible in the region of the mandibular premolars. Radiographically it appears as a small ovoid or round radiolucent area in the region of the premolars. It may also be noted in some cases in the molar region. It should be differentiated from periapical pathology.

Mylohyoid Ridge

The mylohyoid ridge is also called as the internal oblique ridge. It is located on the internal surface of the mandible as a linear prominence. It extends downward and forward from the molar region to the mandibular symphysis. It gives attachment to the mylohyoid muscle. Radiographically it appears as a dense radiopaque band and is most prominent in the molar region. Sometimes it is superimposed over the roots of the mandibular teeth.

Mandibular Canal

The mandibular canal is the largest nutrient canal of the jaws. It extends from the mandibular foramen to the mental foramen and houses the inferior alveolar nerve and blood vessels. In the mandibular periapical radiograph it appears as a thick radiolucent band with radiopaque borders. The radiopaque lines are the cortical walls (Fig. 10-3).

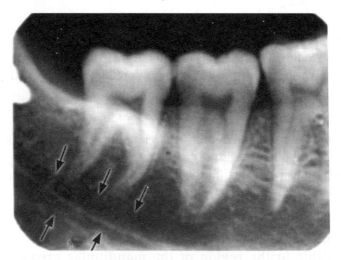

Fig. 10-3: Mandibular canal

External Oblique Ridge

The external oblique ridge extends anteriorly and downward from the anterior border of the ramus of the mandible, on the outer aspect of the alveolar process. It appears as a bony prominence and merges below the first molar. This forms a line of attachment for the buccinator muscle. In the radiograph it appears superior to the internal oblique ridge even though anatomically they have a parallel course.

Submandibular Fossa

The submandibular fossa or the mandibular fossa or the submaxillary fossa is a depressed area located on the internal surface of the mandible, below the mylohyoid ridge. It serves as the site for the submandibular salivary gland. Radiographically it appears as a radiolucent area in the molar region below the mylohyoid ridge.

Coronoid Process

The coronoid process of the mandible, though is a part of the mandible, appears quite often in the intraoral periapical radiograph of the maxillary posterior region as a triangular radiopacity either superimposed over, or inferior to the maxillary tuberosity region.

Chapter 11

Extraoral Radiography

My how or when Thou wilt not heed,
But come down Thine own secret stair,
That Thou mayst answer all my need—
Yes, every bygone prayer.

– George Macdonald

INTRODUCTION

Due to the smaller size of the film, *intraoral* radiographs have the limitation of not providing adequate diagnostic information. Intraoral radiographs also are not very useful in the diagnosis of any pathology or trauma involving the skull and the facial bones. In these situations, extraoral radiographs are necessary for arriving at a diagnosis.

PURPOSE OF EXTRAORAL RADIOGRAPHS

- For the evaluation of a larger area of the skull and the jaws
- For the evaluation of growth and development
- In the evaluation of multiple impacted teeth
- To detect any pathology or condition involving the jaws
- To examine the complete extent of a large lesion
- In the evaluation of trauma
- To evaluate the temporomandibular joint (TMJ).

Most of the extraoral radiographs are taken with screen-film combination. The use of intensifying screens effectively reduces the radiation exposure to the patient. Though some extraoral radiographs can be taken with intraoral machines, most of the extraoral radiographs are taken with specialized machines.

LATERAL JAW PROJECTION

Lateral jaw projection is useful to examine the posterior region of the mandible. This radiographic projection is also called as lateral oblique view. This radiograph is very useful in the diagnosis of fracture or any pathology in patients with restricted mouth opening.

Two types of lateral jaw projection are
- Body of the mandible projection
- Ramus of the mandible projection.

Body of the Mandible Projection (Fig. 11-1)

This projection is used in the evaluation of impacted teeth, fracture of the body of the mandible and any pathology (cysts or tumors) involving the mandibular premolar-molar region and inferior border of the mandible.

8 × 10 or 5 × 7 inches screen-film combination is used for this radiographic projection. The film is kept flat against the cheek of the required side and is centered over the body of the mandible. The head is tilted 15 degrees to the side being imaged

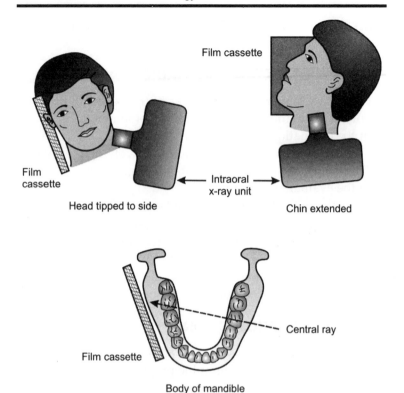

Fig. 11-1: Body of the mandible projection

and the chin is elevated and extended upward. The central x-ray beam is directed perpendicular to the horizontal plane of the cassette with a vertical angulation of -15 to -20 degrees. The x-ray beam should enter at a point centered on the body of the mandible.

Ramus of the Mandible Projection (Fig. 11-2)

In the ramus of the mandible projection, the film is held flat on the cheek of the required side and centered over the ramus of the mandible. The head is tilted 15 degrees towards the required side and the chin is elevated and extended. The central x-ray beam should be perpendicular to the plane of the cassette at a vertical angulation of -15 to -20 degrees and centered on the ramus of the mandible.

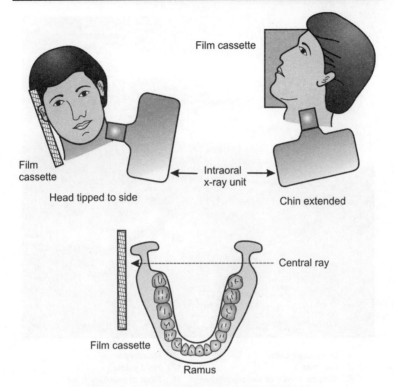

Film cassette

Film cassette

Intraoral x-ray unit

Head tipped to side

Chin extended

Central ray

Film cassette

Ramus

Fig. 11-2: Ramus of the mandible projection

SKULL RADIOGRAPHY

Although some skull radiographs can be taken with intraoral x-ray machines, most require an extraoral unit. Skull radiographs are difficult to interpret because of the superimposition of various anatomic structures. Various skull projections are:
• Lateral cephalometric projection
• Posteroanterior projection (P-A view)
• Waters projection (paranasal sinus or PNS view)
• Submentovertex projection
• Reverse Towne projection.

Lateral Cephalometric Projection (Figs 11-3 and 11-4)

Lateral skull projection or lateral cephalometric projection is popularly known as lateral cephalogram. This radiograph is

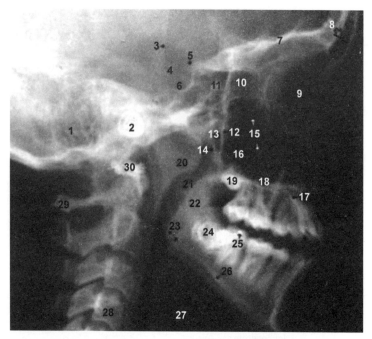

1. Mastoid air cells	16. Maxillary sinus
2. Ear rods	17. Hard palate
3. Anterior border of head positioner	18. Floor of maxillary sinus
4. Posterior clinoid process	19. Developing max 3rd molar
5. Anterior clinoid process	20. Ramus of mandible
6. Sella turcica	21. Nasopharyngeal airspace
7. Floor of anterior cranial vault	22. Soft palate
8. Frontal sinus	23. Oropharyngeal airspace
9. Orbit	24. Developing mand 3rd molar
10. Ethmoid sinus	25. Amalgam restoration
11. Sphenoid sinus	26. Inferior border of mand
12. Posterior wall of max. sinus	27. Hyoid bone
13. Pterygomaxillary fissure	28. Body of 4th cervical vertebra
14. Ptergoid plates	29. Posterior tubercle of atlas
15. Zygoma	30. Ear ring

Fig. 11-3: Lateral skull projection (radiograph)

very useful in the evaluation of facial growth and development, trauma, pathology, and developmental anomalies. This projection shows bones of the skull and the face as well as soft tissue profile of the face.

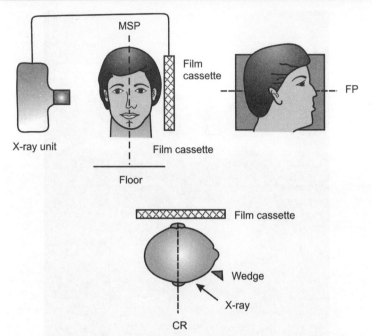

Fig. 11-4: Lateral cephalometric projection (technique)

8 × 10 inches screen-film combination is used for this projection. The cassette is kept perpendicular to the floor. The left side of the patient's head is positioned close to the cassette. The midsagittal plane is perpendicular to the floor and parallel to the cassette. The Frankfort horizontal plane (a line extending from the top of the external auditory meatus to the infraorbital margin) is parallel to the floor. The teeth should be in occlusion and the lips should be gently closed. The central x-ray beam is directed through the center of the cassette. The target to object distance is more, that is, 60 inches.

Posteroanterior Projection (Figs 11-5A and B)

Posteroanterior projection or PA view is used in the evaluation of facial growth and development, trauma, any pathology and developmental anomalies. This projection demonstrates the frontal and ethmoidal sinuses, the orbits and the nasal cavity.

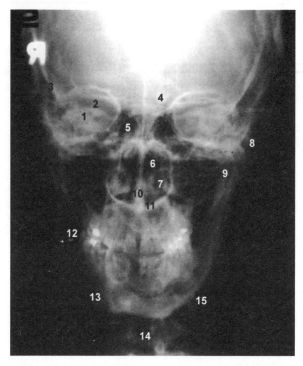

1. Petrous portion of temporal bone
2. Orbit
3. Innominate bone
4. Frontal sinus
5. Sphenoid and ethmoid sinuses
6. Middle nasal turbinate
7. Inferior nasal turbinate
8. Mastoid air cells
9. Coronoid process of mandible
10. Nasal septum
11. Floor of nasal fossa/hard palate
12. Mandibular canal
13. Mental foramen
14. Cervical vertebra
15. Soft tissue outline of face

Fig. 11-5A: Posteroanterior view

8 × 10 inches screen-film combination is used and the cassette is placed perpendicular to the floor. The long axis of the cassette is positioned vertically. The patient faces the cassette in such a way that the forehead and the nose touch the surface. Frankfort plane is parallel to the floor.

The central x-ray beam is aligned perpendicular to the center of the head and the cassette.

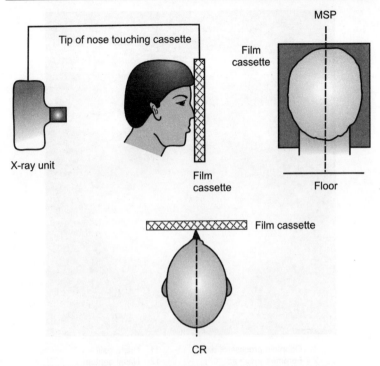

Fig. 11-5B: Patient position for posteroanterior projection

Waters Projection (Figs 11-6A and B)

Waters projection or paranasal sinus projection or PNS projection is used in the evaluation of the maxillary sinus. This projection also demonstrates the frontal and the ethmoid sinuses, the orbits, and the nasal cavity. This projection is very useful in the diagnosis of maxillary sinusitis and fracture of the facial bones (the margins of the orbit and Le Fort II and III fractures). 8 × 10 inches screen-film combination is used and the cassette is placed perpendicular to the floor. The long axis of the cassette is placed in a vertical direction.

The patient faces the cassette with the chin touching the cassette. The tip of the nose is positioned 1/2 to 1 inch away from the cassette. The midsagittal plane is perpendicular to the floor and the head is positioned on the center of the cassette. The central x-ray beam is directed from the center of the head.

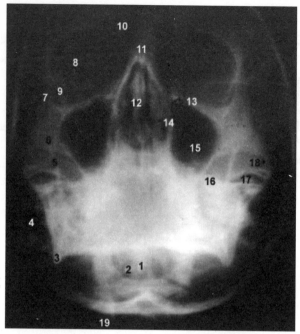

1. Odontoid process of axis	11. Crista galli
2. Foramen magnum	12. Nasal septum
3. Angle of mandible	13. Ethmoid air cells
4. Mastoid air cells	14. Nasal turbinates
5. Coronoid process of mand.	15. Maxillary sinus
6. Body of zygoma	16. Petrous ridge
7. Frontal process of zygoma	17. Mandibular fossa
8. Orbit	18. Zygomatic arch
9. Innominate line	19. Cervical vertebra
10. Frontal sinus	

Fig. 11-6A: Waters projection

Submentovertex Projection (Figs 11-7 and 11-8)

The submentovertex view (SMV) helps to identify the position of the condyle, visualize base of the skull, and evaluate fractures of the zygomatic arch. This projection also demonstrates the sphenoid and the ethmoid sinuses and lateral wall of the maxillary sinus.

Submentovertex view is of two types:
• Zygomatic arch projection
• Base of the skull projection.

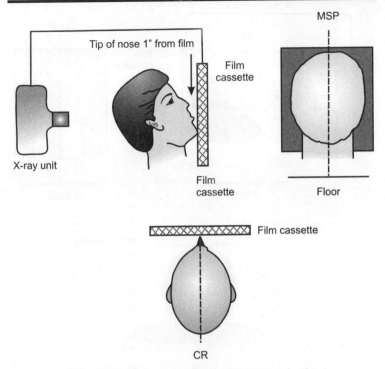

Fig. 11-6B: Patient position for Waters projection

Zygomatic Arch Projection

Zygomatic arch projection is also called as the jug handle view. This radiograph is essentially similar to base of the skull projection with the exception that the radiation exposure and development time are less to prevent overexposure and resultant blackout of the zygomatic arch.

Base of the Skull Projection

For both zygomatic arch projection and base of the skull projection, 8 × 10 inches screen-film combination is used. The cassette is placed perpendicular to the floor with the long axis vertical.

The patient's head and neck are extended backwards as far as possible. The vertex or top of the skull touches the cassette. The midsagittal plane and the Frankfort plane are positioned

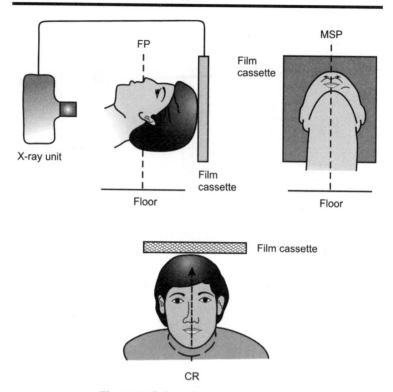

Fig. 11-7: Submentovertex projection

perpendicular to the floor. The head is centered on the cassette. The central x-ray beam is directed through the center of the head and perpendicular to the center of the cassette.

Another method of taking this radiograph is by using dental x-ray machine used for intraoral radiography. The patient is asked to sit on the dental chair used for intraoral radiography. The head and neck are tipped backward in such a way that the midsagittal plane is perpendicular to the floor. The cassette is placed in such a way that the vertex is touching the plane of the cassette and is held vertically. The intraoral x-ray cone is placed in the submental region so that the central x-ray beam enters at a midpoint in the submandibular region and is directed through the center of the head and perpendicular to the cassette.

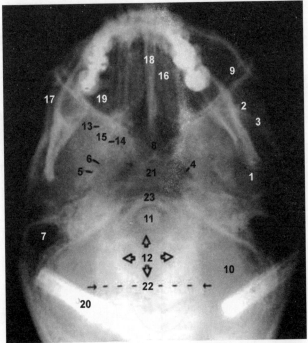

1. Mandibular condyle
2. Coronoid process of mandible
3. Anterior wall of middle cranial fossa
4. Carotid canal
5. Foramen spinosum
6. Foramen ovale
7. Mastoid air cells
8. Sphenoid sinus
9. Lateral wall of maxillary sinus
10. Posterior cranial fossa
11. Odontoid process of axis
12. Foramen magnum
13. Lateral pterygoid plate
14. Medial pterygoid plate
15. Pterygoid fossa
16. Ethmoid sinus
17. Zygoma
18. Nasal septum
19. Maxillary sinus
20. Hair clip
21. Pharynx
22. Vertebrae
23. Arch of C-1

Fig. 11-8: Submentovertex projection

Reverse Towne Projection (Fig. 11-9)

Reverse Towne projection helps in the identification of fractures involving the condylar neck and the ramus area.

This projection is made with 8 × 10 inches screen-film combination. The cassette is placed perpendicular to the floor with the long axis vertically aligned.

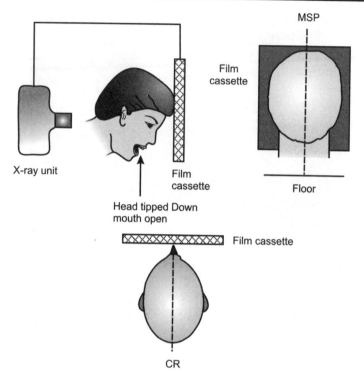

Fig. 11-9: Reverse Towne projection

The patient faces the cassette and the head is tipped down with the mouth in wide open position. The chin almost rests on the chest, whereas the top of the forehead touches the cassette. The midsagittal plane is perpendicular to the floor. The central x-ray beam is directed through the center of the head to the center of the cassette.

TEMPOROMANDIBULAR JOINT (TMJ) VIEWS

The bony elements forming the TMJ are the glenoid fossa of the temporal bone, the mandibular condyle and the articular eminence of the temporal bone. The articular disk is present between the bony elements, thus dividing the joint space into an upper and a lower compartments.

Radiography of the TMJ is not very successful because of the proximity of several bony structures. Another important disadvantage of TMJ radiography is that, most of the TMJ-related complaints may have a soft tissue component with the result that radiographs do not play much role in the diagnosis.

The various TMJ views are:
- Transcranial view
- Transorbital view
- Transpharyngeal view
- TMJ tomography.

Transcranial View (Fig. 11-10)

Transcranial projection helps in the visualization of the superior surface of the condyle and the articular eminence. The joint space is also visualized.

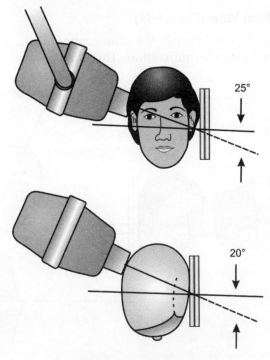

Fig. 11-10: Transcranial projection

This projection can be made either with 5 × 7 inches or 8 × 10 inches screen-film combination. Projections are made separately for each joint.

The cassette is placed flat over the ear of the required side in such a way that it is centered over the TMJ. The midsagittal plane is perpendicular to the floor and parallel with the cassette. The central x-ray beam is directed to a point 2 inches superior to and 0.5 inch behind the opening of the ear canal (external auditory meatus). The central x-ray beam is directed downward by 25 degrees and forward by 20 degrees and centered on the TMJ to be radiographed. This projection can be made by using intraoral x-ray machine.

There are special positioning devices available to standardize the procedure. This helps in comparing the right and left TMJ at the same time and under standardized conditions.

Transorbital View (Fig. 11-11) *Zimmer, Transmaüilbary*

Transorbital view helps in the visualization of the joint with relatively less superimposition. This view is also called as

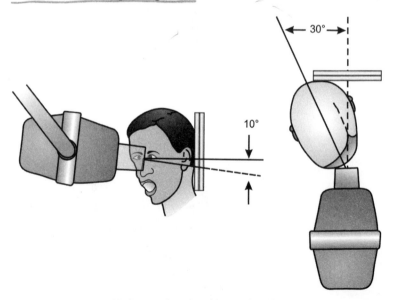

Fig. 11-11: Transorbital projection

Zimmer projection or transmaxillary projection. This view demonstrates the entire lateromedial articulating surfaces of both the condyle and the articular eminence and the condylar neck.

This projection is made either by using 5 × 7 inches or 8 × 10 inches screen-film combination. Separate projections are made for the left and right sides.

In the sitting position, the head of the patient is tipped down about 10 degrees in such a way that the canthomeatal line is horizontal. The midsagittal plane is kept at 30 degrees to the central x-ray beam by moving the head to the left for left side projection and to the right for right side projection. The cassette is positioned behind the patient's head and the central x-ray beam is directed through the ipsilateral orbit and through the required TMJ, exiting from the skull behind the mastoid process. During the exposure, the patient is asked to open the mouth as wide as possible.

Transpharyngeal View (Fig. 11-12)

Transpharyngeal projection is also called as infracranial view, Parma projection, or McQueen projection. This projection

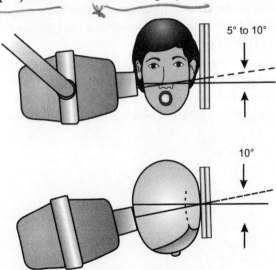

Fig. 11-12: Transpharyngeal projection

demonstrates the condylar process from the midmandibular ramus to the condyle. This technique helps in the diagnosis of fractures of the condyle and the condylar neck and in detecting alterations in the condylar morphology.

This projection is made with 5 × 7 or 8 × 10 inches screen-film combination. The cassette is held over the ear in such a way that the TMJ of interest is within the center of the cassette. The cassette is held parallel to the midsagittal plane. The x-ray tube is kept on the side of the skull opposite to the TMJ imaged. It is angled in such a way that the central beam is directed cranially 5–10 degrees and posteriorly approximately 10 degrees. Before the exposure, the patient is asked to open the mouth wide so that the central x-ray beam enters through the tubeside sigmoid notch, below the skull base, oropharynx, and through the TMJ of the filmside in an oblique direction to the long axis of the condyle.

Temporomandibular Joint Tomography

Tomography is a technique used to demonstrate structures located within a particular plane while blurring out structures outside this plane. In TMJ tomography this is accomplished by moving the film and the x-ray tubehead in opposite directions around a rotation point.

Tomography helps in the visualization of the condyle, the articular eminence, and the glenoid fossa. It can also be used to determine the joint space and to evaluate the extent of movement of the condyle when the mouth is opened.

Chapter 12

Panoramic Radiography

- *Introduction*
- *Purpose and Uses*
- *Disadvantages*
- *Fundamental Principles of Panoramic Radiography*
- *Technique*

Stood forth in the tempest of doubt and disaster,
Unaided, and single, the danger to brave,
Asserted thy claims, and the rights of his master,
Preserved thee to conquer, and saved thee to save.

– Thomas Babbington Macaulay

INTRODUCTION

Panoramic radiography is a specialized extraoral radiographic technique used to examine the upper and the lower jaws in a single film. Panoramic radiography is also called as rotational panoramic radiography or pantomography.

In this technique, the film and the tube head (x-ray source) rotate around the patient who remains stationary and produce a series of individual images successively in a single film. As these images are combined in a single film, overall view of the maxilla, the mandible and related structures is obtained.

Purpose and Uses

- For visualizing the maxilla and the mandible in one film
- For patient education

- To evaluate impacted teeth
- In the evaluation of multiple unerupted supernumerary teeth
- To evaluate eruption sequence and pattern, growth and development
- To detect any pathology involving the jaws
- To examine the extent of a large lesion
- To evaluate traumatic injuries
- For radiographic examination of patients with limited mouth opening
- To identify diseases of the temporomandibular joint
- In the evaluation of elongated styloid process.

Disadvantages

There are some obvious disadvantages of a panoramic view in spite of its valuable use. These are the following:

- Images in a panoramic film are not as sharp as in an intraoral film or the resolution is very low.
- Panoramic radiography cannot be used in the diagnosis of caries
- Panoramic radiography cannot be used in the evaluation of bone loss due to periodontal disease
- Panoramic radiographic image shows superimposition, especially in the premolar region
- Structures in the anterior region may not be well-defined
- Structures outside the image layer cannot be visualized
- Panoramic radiography cannot be used as a substitute for intraoral radiography.

Fundamental Principles of Panoramic Radiography

Panoramic radiography is based on the principle of tomography and scanography.

Tomography is defined as an unobstructed view of a structure in different directions without interference from structures above or below that plane. In other words, tomography is a radiographic technique, which allows the imaging of one layer or section of the body while blurring out the images from structures in other planes (Fig. 12-1).

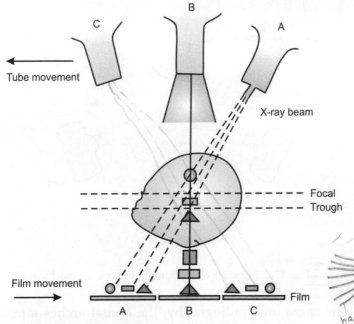

Fig. 12-1: Diagrammatic representation of tomography

Scanography or narrow beam radiography or slit beam radiography refers to a narrow beam of radiation successively scanning different areas of the patient's tissues to cast image in a single film.

In this technique, the cassette carrier and the x-ray tube head are connected and rotate around a patient during exposure. As the cassette carrier rotates around the patient, it also rotates in such a way as to cast image from one end of the film to the other. The axis or pivotal point around which the cassette carrier and the x-ray tube head rotate is the 'rotation center' (Fig. 12-2). The different types of rotation centers used by different manufacturers are the following:

1. Double-rotation center
2. Triple-rotation center
3. Continuously moving rotation center.

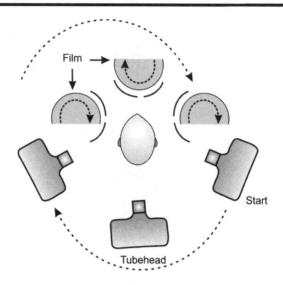

Fig. 12-2: Principle of working of panoramic machine

In panoramic radiography, the dental arches must be positioned near to the focal trough to achieve the clearest image. The focal trough is defined as a three-dimensional curved zone in which structures are clearly demonstrated in a panoramic radiograph (Fig. 12-3). The structures located inside or outside the focal trough appear blurred or indistinct. In the panoramic machines, the focal trough is narrow in the anterior region and wide in the posterior region.

Functionally, the panoramic x-ray tube head is similar to the intraoral x-ray tube head. The collimator of the tube head differs in that it permits only a narrow beam to pass through. The unit has a head positioner (containing chin rest, notched bite-block, forehead rest, and lateral head supporter). Screen-film combination is used in panoramic radiography. Flexible cassette is used for adaptation to the curved cassette carrier. The cassette must be marked 'R' and 'L' to orient the film. In some machines rigid cassettes are used.

A panoramic radiograph is unique as the focus of projection in the horizontal dimension is different from the vertical projection. In the horizontal dimension the rotation center is

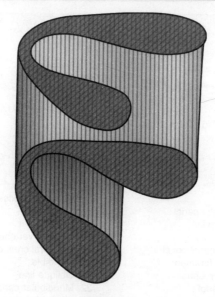

Fig. 12-3: Focal trough

the functional focus, whereas in the vertical dimension the x-ray source serves as the focus.

Panoramic radiograph has definite and serious disadvantage. This is due to the appearance of "ghost image". Ghost image is a radiopaque artifact seen in a panoramic film that is produced when a radiodense object is penetrated twice by the x-ray beam. A ghost image resembles the real image. However, it is seen on the opposite side of the film, it is indistinct, larger, and located at a higher level than the real image. To avoid the occurrence of ghost image, the patient should be asked to remove all dense objects from the head and neck region.

Technique

The patient is asked to stand erect. The vertebral column must be straight to avoid superimposition in the radiographic image. The patient is asked to bite on a bite-block. The upper and lower teeth are placed in an edge-to-edge position to align close to the focal trough. The midsagittal plane is perpendicular to the

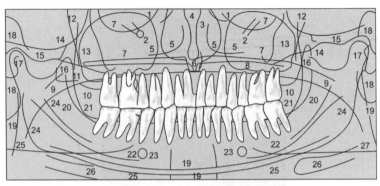

1. Orbit	16. Coronoid process
2. Infraorbital canal	17. Condyle
3. Nasal cavity	18. External ear
4. Nasal septum	19. Cervical vertebrae
5. Inferior nasal concha	20. Temporal crest of the
6. Incisive foramen	mandible
7. Maxillary sinus	21. Oblique line
8. Palatal roof	22. Mandibular canal
9. Soft palate	23. Mental foramen
10. Maxillary tuberosity	24. Dorsum of the tongue
11. Pterygoid processes	25. Inferior border of the
12. Pterygopalatine fossa	mandible
13. Zygomatic bone	26. Hyoid bone
14. Zygomaticotemporal suture	27. Superimposition of the
15. Zygomatic arch	contralateral jaw.

Fig. 12-4: Structures visualized in a panoramic radiograph

floor. The patient's head must not be bent or tilted. An imaginary line extending from the infraorbital margin to the center of the external auditory meatus should be parallel to the floor. The tongue should touch the palate during exposure. The patient should remain still during the exposure. The film processing is similar to other radiographic film processing. (Fig. 12-4) shows various structures visualized in a panoramic radiograph.

Chapter 13

Localization Technique

- *Introduction*
- *Right-angle Technique*
- *Tube Shift Principle*
- *Definition and Evaluation*
- *Pantomography*

"But while Oppression lifts its head,
Or a tyrant would be lord,
Though we may thank him for the plough,
We'll never forget the sword!"

– **Charles Mackay**

INTRODUCTION

A radiograph is a two-dimensional representation (image) of a three-dimensional structure (object) in the superoinferior and anteroposterior plane. In many clinical situations proper localization is necessary for diagnosis and further management.

The localization technique is used to derive three-dimensional information from two-dimensional images. This objective is achieved by making use of usually two radiographs.

Some indications for resorting to localization technique are:
- To establish the position of structures in the buccolingual plane (e.g. impacted teeth)
- To determine displacement of fracture
- For tracking of broken needles and instruments

- For localizing foreign objects
- In localizing displaced root in the maxillary sinus
- For differentiating buccal and palatal roots as well as additional root canals in endodontic practice
- To determine root positions
- In the detection of salivary gland stone
- In the evaluation of restorative materials.

There are four techniques, which are employed in the localization. These techniques are the following:
1. Right-angle technique
2. Tube shift principle
3. Definition evaluation
4. Pantomography.

RIGHT-ANGLE TECHNIQUE

The right-angle technique is sometimes called as Miller's right angle technique. This technique helps in the orientation of structures seen in the radiographs. This technique uses two radiographic projections taken at right angles to each other. First, a periapical film is exposed using proper technique to show the position of the object in the superoinferior and anteroposterior relationship. Then, an occlusal film is exposed directing the central x-ray beam perpendicular to the film. The occlusal film represents the object in buccolingual and anteroposterior relationships. The two radiographs are compared for locating the object in three-dimension.

This technique can be effectively used in locating maxillary impacted canine (with periapical projection and maxillary occlusal projection) or in case of fracture of the mandible, to locate any displacement (with orthopantomogram or lateral oblique projection and mandibular occlusal projection).

TUBE SHIFT PRINCIPLE

The tube shift principle is also called as the buccal object rule or Clark's rule (named after CA Clark who proposed the technique in 1910). The principle of this technique is that relative position of radiographic images of two separate objects changes when the projection angle at which the images were made, is changed (Fig. 13-1). This technique uses a different horizontal angulation to locate vertically aligned images or to locate the object in the buccal aspect or lingual aspect with reference to a reference structure.

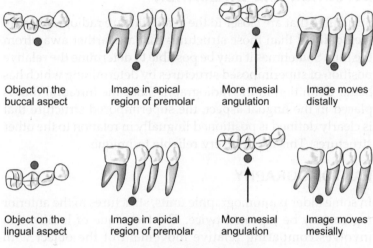

| Object on the buccal aspect | Image in apical region of premolar | More mesial angulation | Image moves distally |

| Object on the lingual aspect | Image in apical region of premolar | More mesial angulation | Image moves mesially |

Fig. 13-1: Tube shift principle

To determine the relative buccolingual relationship between two structures that appear to be superimposed, a second radiograph is taken with the tube shifted about 20 degrees either mesially or distally. The point of entry of the x-ray beam, film position and vertical angulation remain the same as in the first projection. When the two radiographs are compared, the object present on the buccal aspect seems to be moving in the opposite direction of the projection angle in the second radiograph and the object present on the lingual aspect seems to be moving in the same direction as the changed projection angle with reference to the reference structure. If there is no change in the radiographic image with the changed projection angle, the object is located in the same vertical plane as the reference structure.

This technique can be easily remembered by a mnemonic SLOB (Same-Lingual, Opposite-Buccal). If the image of the object moves in the same direction with reference to the reference structure, the object is lingually placed and if the image of the object moves in the opposite direction with reference to the reference structure, the object is buccally placed.

DEFINITION AND EVALUATION

Structures that are closer to the x-ray film are radiographically well-defined than those structures that are farther away from the film. Sometimes it may be possible to determine the relative position of superimposed structures by determining which has better definition in the radiograph. Since the intraoral film is placed in the lingual aspect, the superimposed structure that is clearly defined is positioned lingually in relation to the other structures. This is not a very reliable technique.

PANTOMOGRAPHY

In some older pantomographic units, structures in the anterior region may be repeated twice. The technique of localization involves comparing relative movement of the object with adjacent structures from one side of the film to the other with the direction that the clinician views the film (e.g. left to right). If the object is present lingually, it seems to be moving in the same direction as the clinician's viewing movement and in the opposite direction if it is present on the buccal side.

Chapter 14

Specialized Radiographs in Dental Radiology

- *Xeroradiography*
- *Sialography*
- *Conventional Tomography*
- *Computerized Tomography*
- *Magnetic Resonance Imaging*
- *Ultrasound Technique*
- *Nuclear Medicine*
- *Thermography*
- *Arthrography*
- *Radiovisiography*
- *Digital Panoramic Radiography*

For heathen heart that puts her trust
In reeking tube and iron shard—
    All valiant dust that builds on dust,
And guarding, calls not Thee to guard—
    For frantic boast and foolish word,
Thy mercy on Thy people, Lord!
    Amen.

– Rudyard Kipling

XERORADIOGRAPHY

As the name implies, xeroradiography is a specialized radiographic technique, which does not make use of the wet processing technique of the image receptor after being exposed to x-rays. The principal difference between xeroradiography and conventional radiography is that, in xeroradiography, the image formation is achieved by a photoelectrostatic process and not by photochemical process as in conventional radiography.

Xeroradiography has found its application in the medical field in the early part of 1950s. Xeroradiography uses certain materials such as selenium that are photoconductors or semiconductors and conduct electric current when they interact with electromagnetic radiations such as light or x-rays.

In xeroradiography, selenium-coated aluminium plate is used as the image receptor system. Sensitivity of selenium is achieved by coating it with a uniform charge. The charged plate is placed in a lightproof cassette and exposed to x-rays as in the case of conventional radiography. When the x-ray photons strike the plate there will be discharge in the plates, which is proportional to the intensity of the beam striking the area. Thus, any alteration in the intensity of the x-ray beam as it passes through the object results in different degrees of discharge. This results in the formation of an electrostatic charge pattern. This image is developed by passing oppositely charged toner particles over the plate (Fig. 14-1). These particles get attracted

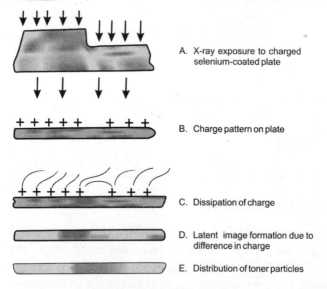

A. X-ray exposure to charged selenium-coated plate

B. Charge pattern on plate

C. Dissipation of charge

D. Latent image formation due to difference in charge

E. Distribution of toner particles

Fig. 14-1: Xeroradiography

to variably charged areas depending on the intensity of the remaining charge. This image formed by the toner particles is fused to paper or laminated between a transparent and a translucent sheet of plastic. The first type of image can be viewed by reflected light, whereas the second type of image can be viewed by reflected or transmitted light.

The charging and processing are done automatically in a light-tight processor and requires only electric current. The entire procedure requires only 20–90 seconds. The plates can be reused for about 1000 times.

Advantages of Xeroradiography

- No necessity of handling wet film as in conventional radiography
- No requirement of darkroom
- No requirement of plumbing
- No requirement of processing solution and replenisher
- The process is faster
- Dry and permanent image is formed
- The plates can be used for about 1000 exposures. Therefore, it is cost effective
- The image has a broader recording latitude
- Visible image of air, fat, water, cartilage, and bone can be seen
- Images have good detail or edge enhancement (exaggeration of boundaries between areas of differing radiodensities due to increased deposition of the toner particles at the highly charged area and decreased deposition at the lower-charged area)
- Xeroradiograph has better resolution
- Xeroradiographic image has less granularity (good image quality)
- The technique requires less radiation exposure.

SIALOGRAPHY

The examination of the salivary glands often faces considerable difficulty due to the lack of direct access for visual as well as exploratory examination. Though a good deal of information can be obtained based on the history and clinical examination, the diagnostic procedure is incomplete without the specialized radiographic examination called sialography.

Sialography is the radiographic visualization of the ductal tree of the parotid or submandibular salivary glands by means of the intraductal injection of a radiopaque contrast solution to delineate the ductal pattern which will be radiographically discernible.

Sialography may be performed to determine the functional capacity of the salivary gland, to determine any obstruction, in the diagnosis of intraglandular neoplasm, in case of facial swellings to rule out neoplasm of the salivary gland, for the forceful removal of mucous plugs, or for the antiinflammatory action brought about by the iodine-based contrast agent.

Hypersensitivity to the contrast agent and acute infections (e.g. acute parotitis) are contraindications for sialography. The allergic reactions are more often associated with fat-soluble contrast agents. Sialography has been shown to aggravate acute infections.

The procedure of sialography requires the following instruments:
- A set of graded lacrimal probes
- Cannula or 18–22 gauge needle
- 5 ml syringe
- Contrast agent
- Facility for radiographic examination without any delay.

The contrast agents used in sialography can be broadly divided into fat-soluble (e.g. Lipiodol) and water-soluble (e.g. Hypaque, Renografin, Conray 210, and Conray 420) contrast agents. As the fat-soluble contrast agents are more viscous, it is easy for handling and the contrast will be more intense. The water-soluble contrast agents do not cause much patient discomfort or hypersensitivity reaction and fill finer elements of the duct. The contrast brought about by water-soluble contrast agents will be less intense.

The procedure involves introduction of the contrast agent through the duct opening after enlarging it by using graded lacrimal probes. Before the procedure, the patient should be asked to rinse the mouth with an antiseptic solution. The amount of contrast agent required for submandibular sialography is about 0.5–1.2 ml and for parotid sialography, 0.8–2 ml. The contrast agent is introduced until the patient feels discomfort or fullness in the gland area. A radiograph is taken immediately thereafter. The radiographs taken for parotid sialography are either anteroposterior view or orthopantomogram. The radiographs taken for submandibular sialography are either lateral oblique view, lateral skull projection, mandibular occlusal view, orthopantomogram, or anteroposterior view.

After taking a suitable radiograph, the patient is asked to suck on a lemon or 1% citric acid to induce saliva secretion. Another radiograph is taken after 30 minutes. A normal salivary gland excretes the contrast agent within 30 minutes.

A properly done sialogram may not be difficult to interpret. There are various radiographic appearances of sialogram depending on the pathology. A normal sialogram is described as having branched leafless tree or naked tree appearance. In case of stones within the duct, there will be filling defect distal to the site of obstruction. There can also be dilatation of the duct proximal to the obstruction. Intraglandular neoplasm may give the so-called 'ball-in-hand' appearance. Autoimmune disorders (e.g. Sjögren's syndrome) result in thinning of individual ducts and decrease in the number of ducts. The typical sialographic appearance is called 'cherry-blossom' or branchless fruit-laden tree appearance.

CONVENTIONAL TOMOGRAPHY

Tomography is a process of visualization of a layer within the body without interference from structures above and below that layer (Fig. 14-2). This objective is achieved by moving the x-ray tube and the film around a fulcrum (center of rotation)

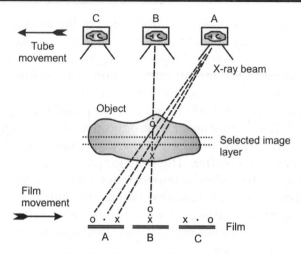

Fig. 14-2: Principle of tomography

and the objects that are closer to the point of rotation are defined clearly and the objects farthest away from the point of rotation are blurred. The thickness of the image layer depends on the movement of the x-ray tube and the angle of rotation. If the movement along the path is small, the image layer becomes thick. On the other hand if the path of movement or the angle is increased, the image layer decreases (Fig. 14-3). The blurring is more at the periphery of the image layer and sharpest image is seen at the center.

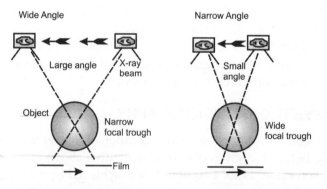

Fig. 14-3: Variability in the thickness of the image layer

Different patterns of movement of the x-ray tube and the film are linear, circular, trispiral, elliptical, and hypocycloidal (Fig. 14-4). Apart from these, there are other multidirectional movements also. Tomography has found its application in dental radiology in the visualization of the temporomandibular joint and other facial structures.

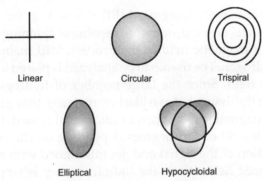

Linear   Circular   Trispiral

Elliptical   Hypocycloidal

Fig. 14-4: Different tomographic movements

COMPUTERIZED TOMOGRAPHY

Computerized tomography (CT) has a prominent role in the medical imaging. In this technique x-ray scanning and digital computer technology are used successfully to achieve the required goal. With the help of CT scan, the required structure can be clearly visualized without any superimposition. In this technique, the object to be visualized is divided into a series of sections or slices and each section is scanned several times and from many different angles. The x-ray beam coming out of the section is received by radiation detectors.

The x-ray attenuation characteristics of the different sections in different angles are processed by a digital computer. The computer constructs the density profile.

CT scanning is very efficient in the discrimination of different densities, even of less than 10%. Thus CT scanning can be used to study normal blood, clotted blood, cerebrospinal fluid (CSF), brain tumors, normal soft tissues, and neoplasms. CT scanning is very useful in the diagnosis of intracranial lesions and in the evaluation of traumatic injuries. Considering the depth of information obtained, the radiation exposure to the patient is also very less.

MAGNETIC RESONANCE IMAGING

Magnetic resonance imaging (MRI) is based on the principle that the nuclei of some atoms are capable of spinning and they generate a magnetic field in the process. MRI mainly makes use of hydrogen. The tissues to be analyzed is placed in a strong magnetic field. Since the large number of hydrogen atoms present in the tissues behave like tiny magnets, they get aligned with the magnetic field. When a radio signal is used, these tiny magnets flip 90 or 180 degrees depending on the amplitude and duration of the signal and get misaligned with respect to the magnetic field. When the radiofrequency is stopped, the nuclear magnets relax and flip back in alignment with the magnetic field. As these nuclei relax, they transmit a radio signal whose frequency is unique to the element and a signal strength that is indicative of the element's abundance. An image or MR image is constructed by a computer using these radio signals.

MRI can be used to diagnose lesions not revealed by CT scan. MRI is useful in discriminating malignant tissue from normal tissue. Currently MRI is used to study the skull, chest, abdomen, pelvis, and extremities.

MRI causes malfunction of pacemakers and causes heating and torque of metallic implants.

ULTRASOUND TECHNIQUE

Ultrasound refers to sound waves that are above the range of audible sound waves. This technique employs physical form of energy and not electromagnetic radiation and is based on the principle that sound waves with certain frequency can be reflected by body tissues and can be used as an information carrier for imaging. A pulse of ultrasound when directed into the body, a microphone at the surface listens for the reflected energy or echo. The depth of the reflecting object from the surface is proportional to the time required for the sound to travel to the object and then back to the surface. The location of the reflecting object is determined based on the direction in which the sound generating and the sound listening devices are aimed. These echoes are used to create an image as the amount of energy reflected depends on the density of the object.

Bone and air cannot be imaged by ultrasound because of their high reflective capability and subsequent distortion of the sound. Ultrasound has very useful application in ophthalmology, obstetrics and gynecology, cardiac diseases, and abdominal diseases. It may also be useful in the diagnosis of benign and malignant lesions, inflammatory and cystic lesions as well as in the study of lymph nodes.

NUCLEAR MEDICINE

In nuclear medicine, radioactive compounds are used to study certain tissues (target tissues), to which these compounds have affinities. Nuclear medicine is a diagnostic radiation science. The various radioactive compounds used in nuclear medicine are also called as radionuclides or radioactive nuclides. A nuclide refers to a species of atom having in its nucleus a particular number of protons and neutrons. Accordingly, hydrogen has three nuclides, ordinary hydrogen or protium, heavy hydrogen or deuterium, and tritium.

The radioactive substances may be radioactive elements or compounds such as 18F-, 113mIn+++, 99mTcO4, or they may be nonradioactive carrier compounds labeled with a radioisotope such as 67Ga-labeled citrate, 99mTc-labeled polyphosphate, or 125I-labeled human serum albumin.

The radioactive compounds are injected into the body and their concentration in the target tissues is detected by external detectors and imaging systems.

Using the radionuclides, the study of various organs or tissues depends on:

• Uptake by an organ
• Excretion
• Dilution.

99mTc is used in the study of the thyroid and the salivary glands. 99Tc is used for "bone scan". Labeling sulfur-colloid with 99mTc can be used to study the reticuloendothelial cells in the liver and the spleen. Cyanocobalamin labeled with 57Co or 60Co is used in Schilling's test. ← Vit B₁₂ · ferrit

Apart from the diagnostic aspects, the radionuclides can also be used in therapy. Some examples are treatment of hyperthyroidism, thyroid cancer, etc.

THERMOGRAPHY

Thermography is a generic title for various methods of quantifying the temperature distribution from body surfaces. There are three forms of thermography used in medical science. They are:
• Liquid crystal thermography (LCT)
• Infrared thermography (IRT)
• Microwave thermography (MCT).

LCT uses cholesterol compounds showing color changes with changes in temperature. MCT and IRT allow the detection of thermal emission from a surface in the microwave and infrared regions of the electromagnetic spectrum. Though still under trial, thermography may find its application in oral inflammatory conditions, screening of oral cancer, management of burns/wound healing, and in the characterization of craniomandibular disorders; particularly temporomandibular joint dysfunction.

ARTHROGRAPHY

In arthrography, contrast agents are introduced into the joint spaces and then radiographed. Water-soluble or fat-soluble contrast agents are used. Arthrography is contraindicated in the presence of infections in or near a joint and in patients who are allergic to the contrast agents.

Separate injections are required for the upper and the lower joint compartments. The needle insertion into the joint space is monitored by fluoroscope.

Arthrography may reveal soft tissue changes not visualized in conventional radiographs such as fibrosis, alteration in the structure of the disk, scarring and fibrosis of the capsule following trauma, and as part of evaluation after TMJ surgery (to visualize silastic implants).

RADIOVISIOGRAPHY

Radiovisiography or RVG refers to a rapid, low-dose, digital imaging system using a small intraoral sensor instead of radiographic film by making use of a charge-coupled device. It presents the possibility of reduced patient exposure and minimal distortion, although resolution and latitude are inferior to standard dental radiography. A receiver or an image-capturing device or a sensor is placed in the mouth and is exposed to x-rays. The signals are then routed to a computer which images the signals on a screen or in print.

The main advantages of using this technique is that the radiation exposure to the patient is minimal and the image is seen almost instantaneously without the requirement of a dark-room or wet-handling of the film. The image thus obtained can also be archived or transferred to a recipient located away.

DIGITAL PANORAMIC RADIOGRAPHY

Digital panoramic radiography is not widely used unlike the conventional panoramic machine. Though the digital system has many distinct adavantages over the conventional panoramic machine, the cost of digital panoramic machine so high. Essentially, the digital panoramic machine has the same principle as that of the RVG system (Fig. 14.5). The panoramic image is captured by a sensor that relays the information to the computer which can be instantly viewed (Fig. 14.6). It is possible to do the digital archiving of the image and it greatly helps in transmitting the image to other locations as image files.

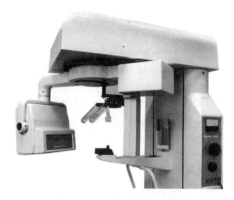

Fig. 14-5: Digital panoramic machine

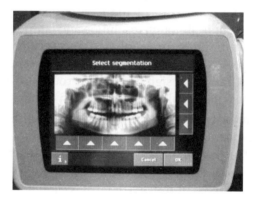

Fig. 14-6: Digital panoramic image

The digital system also makes it easy in the pre- and post-treatment evaluation of the patients. Standard film-based panoramic machines use rare-earth intensifying screens to reduce the amount of radiation required. Depending on the speed of the system, a dose reduction of up to 1/60 can occur compared with direct exposure film. Digital panoramic machines use an electronic detector which is either a CCD or a charge-coupled device which is similar to what is in a digital camera, or a photo-stimulated storage phosphor.

Chapter 15

Radiographic Features of Dental Caries

- *Introduction*
- *Clinical Examination*
- *Radiographic Examination*
- *Classification of Carious Lesions Based on Radiographic Appearance*
- *Radiographic Differential Diagnosis of Dental Caries*

Be good, sweet maid, and let who can be clever;
Do lovely things, not dream them, all day long;
And so make Life, and Death, and that For Ever,
One grand sweet song.

– Charles Kingsley

INTRODUCTION

Dental caries is the destruction of the calcified component of the tooth structure by the action of the acids produced by the oral microorganisms without involving any physical or chemical process. The term caries originates from the Latin word *cariosus*, which means rottenness.

Though most of the dental carious lesions are easily identifiable clinically, radiographs should be supplemented in assessing the depth of the lesions. There are also several occasions wherein caries is diagnosed only through radiographic examination. However, it is prudent to carry out a thorough clinical examination prior to appropriate radiographic examination.

CLINICAL EXAMINATION

The explorer can be used as a tactile device to detect caries. Caries results in 'catches' or 'tug-back' on probing. A progressing caries may also have a 'soft' floor. The color changes of the teeth may not be indicative of tooth decay always. These changes are dark staining in the fissures, pits, and grooves. Smooth surfaces may show chalky white spots or opacity. This is indicative of demineralization process.

RADIOGRAPHIC EXAMINATION

At the site of caries there is a decrease in the density of the tooth material. This facilitates greater penetration of x-rays in these areas. This accounts for the carious lesions appearing as radiolucent in the radiographs.

For effective radiographic diagnosis of dental caries, the radiograph should be free of any technical or processing errors. The radiograph should have good detail and contrast. There should not be any overlapping of proximal surfaces for the detection of proximal caries.

The various radiographs routinely taken for the detection of caries are bitewing and intraoral periapical radiographs.

CLASSIFICATION OF CARIOUS LESIONS BASED ON RADIOGRAPHIC APPEARANCE

Interproximal Caries

Caries occurring between two adjacent teeth is termed interproximal caries. In a radiograph the interproximal caries is usually seen between the contact point and the free gingival margin, in an area called the 'caries susceptible zone'. Radiographically it has a vertical dimension of 1.0–1.5 mm (Fig. 15-1).

The interproximal caries usually has a triangular configuration with the base towards the tooth surface and the apex directed towards the dentinoenamel junction (DEJ). As the caries reaches the DEJ, it spreads laterally and continues into

Contact point

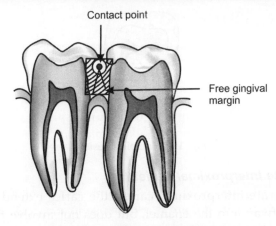

Free gingival
margin

Fig. 15-1: Caries susceptible zone

the dentin. When the caries has invaded the dentin, the base of the triangle is along the DEJ and the apex is directed towards the pulp chamber.

Based on the depth of penetration of caries, interproximal caries can be classified into four types:

Incipient Interproximal Caries

The word incipient means beginning to exist or appear. Radiographically the caries seems to extend less than half the thickness of the enamel (Figs 15-2 and 15-3).

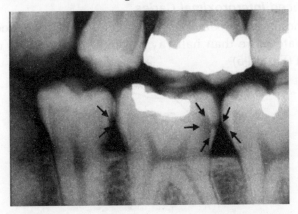

Fig. 15-2: Interproximal caries (see the arrows)

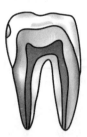

Fig. 15-3: Incipient lesion

Moderate Interproximal Caries

In moderate interproximal caries, the caries extends more than halfway into the enamel, but does not involve the DEJ radiographically. Radiographically, the lesion may appear triangular, diffuse, or combination of the two types (Fig. 15-4).

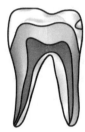

Fig. 15-4: Moderate lesion

Advanced Interproximal Caries

Advanced interproximal caries involves the DEJ, but does not penetrate more than halfway through the thickness of the dentin (Fig. 15-5).

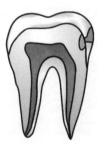

Fig. 15-5: Advanced lesion

Severe Interproximal Caries

Severe interproximal caries has invaded through the thickness of the enamel and has penetrated more than halfway through the thickness of the dentin (Fig. 15-6).

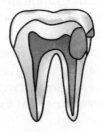

Fig. 15-6: Severe lesion

Occlusal Caries

The occlusal caries begins usually in the pits and fissures of the occlusal surface. Clinical examination is very effective in the detection of occlusal caries and radiographic examination has limited role in the diagnosis. The reason for this limitation is because of the superimposition of the dense buccal and lingual enamel cusps. When the caries involves the DEJ, it may be radiographically evident as a gray shadow.

Occlusal caries can be radiographically classified into the following types.

Incipient Occlusal Caries

Incipient occlusal caries may not be radiographically evident. Clinical examination may reveal a pit on the occlusal surface with a definite 'catch' on probing with an explorer.

Moderate Occlusal Caries

Moderate occlusal caries extends into the dentin and appears as a thin radiolucent line in the radiograph.

Severe Occlusal Caries

Severe occlusal caries extends into the dentin and radiographically appears as a large radiolucency. Clinically this type of lesion is apparent as a large cavitation.

Buccal and Lingual Caries

Buccal caries involves the buccal tooth surface and lingual caries involves the lingual tooth surface. Clinical examination is more useful and important in the diagnosis of buccal and lingual caries because radiographically it may not be always possible to detect caries due to the superimposition of the dense normal tooth structure. It is also not definitely possible to differentiate between buccal and lingual caries based on a radiograph. If at all buccal and lingual caries is radiographically detectable, it appears as a small circular radiolucent area surrounded by dense area of normal tooth structure.

Root Surface Caries

Root surface caries usually begins in the cervical region of the teeth and involves the cementum and the dentin below the cervical region. Usually there is no involvement of the enamel. Some of the predisposing factors for the occurrence of root surface caries are bone loss due to periodontal disease and gingival recession.

Clinical examination alone may not be quite sufficient in the diagnosis of root surface caries, especially in the proximal region. Radiographic examination reveals the extent of involvement of the tooth structure.

On radiographic examination, root surface caries appears as a cupped-out or crater-shaped radiolucency below the cementoenamel junction (CEJ). A root surface caries should be differentiated from cervical burn out.

Recurrent Caries

Secondary or recurrent caries occurs adjacent to a restoration. The predisposing factors for the occurrence of recurrent caries are marginal leakage, defective margins of restoration, fracture of restoration in the marginal region, incomplete removal of caries prior to the placement of filling material, and inadequate cavity preparation or failure to remove complete carious lesion. Recurrent caries radiographically appears as a radiolucent area below or adjacent to a radiopaque restoration. Practically it may be almost impossible to detect recurrent caries adjacent to radiolucent restorative material such as silicate, acrylic and composite.

Rampant Caries

Rampant caries refers to a rapidly spreading type of lesion, affecting many teeth. It usually affects children with poor dietary habits and in adults with poor oral hygiene and decreased saliva flow or with any systemic problems preventing proper maintenance of oral hygiene.

Nursing Bottle Caries

Nursing bottle caries is seen in children who were weaned very early and were given sugar solution as the substitute, especially in the night time. Characteristically, the maxillary anterior teeth are affected and the mandibular anterior teeth are unaffected because of the protective effect of the tongue which covers the mandibular anterior teeth, during feeding from the bottle.

Radiation Caries

Radiotherapy involving the head and neck region with resultant irradiation of the salivary glands causes:
• Decreased saliva secretion
• Increased viscosity of the saliva
• Acidic pH of the saliva
• Loss of buffering capacity of the saliva.

These factors contribute to the development of caries. Three types of radiation caries have been recognized. They are:
  a. One type of radiation caries involves the cementum and dentin in the cervical region of the teeth. It progresses around the teeth
  b. The second type is superficial lesion involving the buccal, occlusal, incisal, and palatal surfaces
  c. The third type appears as dark pigmentation of the entire crown (Fig. 15-7)

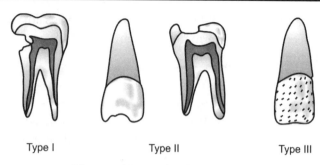

| Type I | Type II | Type III |

Fig. 15-7: Types of radiation caries

RADIOGRAPHIC DIFFERENTIAL DIAGNOSIS OF DENTAL CARIES

It should be stressed that a radiograph should not be relied up on too much in the diagnosis of dental caries. Many radiolucencies on the teeth, as seen in radiographs, may be erroneously diagnosed as caries. A thorough clinical examination should be supplemented with radiographic examination for effective diagnosis of dental caries.

Various other conditions to be considered in the differential diagnosis of dental caries are listed below.

Cervical Burn Out

'Cervical burnout' is a diffuse radiolucent area seen on the mesial or the distal aspects of the teeth in the cervical region between the CEJ and the crest of the alveolar ridge. It is caused by decreased x-ray absorption in this area due to the normal configuration of the affected teeth and also due to 'mach band' effect (an optical illusion as this radiolucent area is contrasted from the radiopaque enamel and the alveolar bone).

Abrasions and Attrition

Radiographically cervical abrasion may resemble caries as there is wearing away of tooth substance resulting in decrease in the density of the involved region. The radiolucency due to abrasion usually produces a well-defined horizontal defect in the cervical region.

In case of attrition, there is wearing away of tooth material in the occlusal or the incisal region. Radiographically attrition is apparent as reduction in the height of the involved teeth or loss of normal 'enamel cap'. Proximal margins of the teeth appear sharp without the usual round contour.

Proximal Wear

Proximal wear is a common phenomenon due to the mesial migration of the teeth. If there is loss of enamel structure due to proximal wear, it may mimic caries as seen in the radiograph.

Indirect Pulp Capping

Often a radiolucent shadow may be seen under a metallic restoration. It is quite common that this radiolucent area may be mistaken for recurrent or secondary caries.

Restorative Materials

Some restorative materials are radiolucent. Restorative materials such as silicate, acrylic, and some composites may resemble caries in the radiographs. However, it may be possible to differentiate between radiolucent restorative material and caries based on the regular geometric outline of a cavity preparation and sometimes the presence of radiopaque cement base. All base materials such as zinc oxyphosphate, zinc oxide, and calcium hydroxide appear radiopaque.

Chapter 16

Radiographic Features of Periodontal Disease

Ghostly it grows, and darker, the burning
Fades into smoke, and now the gusty oaks are
A silent army of phantoms thronging
A land of shadows.

– John Masefield

INTRODUCTION

The term periodontal disease includes gingivitis and periodontitis. Gingivitis refers to the inflammation of the gingiva without involvement of the underlying bone. In many cases gingivitis is due to the deposition of local irritants around the gingival margin and the organisms responsible are nonspecific. The specific organisms that can cause gingivitis are fusospirochetes (*Borrelia vincentii*). *Streptococcus* species, and

Herpes simplex virus. Though periodontitis occurs as a sequela of gingivitis, it is multifactorial in origin. Periodontitis involves the tissues of the periodontium (gingiva, periodontal ligament, alveolar bone, and cementum).

USE OF RADIOGRAPHS IN THE DIAGNOSIS OF PERIODONTAL DISEASE

Radiographs play a vital role in the diagnosis of periodontal disease in the identification of the following initiating factors and status of the periodontium.

- Identifying calculus
- Identifying poorly contoured restorations
- Identifying overextended restorations
- Determining the occlusion
- Determining the root length
- Determining the morphology of the roots
- Determining the crown-root ratio
- Determining the width of the periodontal ligament space
- Evaluation of the condition of the alveolar bone
- Evaluation of the extent of bone loss
- Identification of the furcation involvement
- Evaluation of the number of teeth involved
- Determining the pattern of bone loss
- Determining the location and proximity of the maxillary sinus
- Evaluation of the status of the adjacent teeth
- For proper treatment planning.

It should be kept in mind that the radiographs should be used only as a supplementary diagnostic aid. The importance of clinical examination should never be surpassed by being too much dependent on the radiographs. As the radiograph is a two-dimensional representation of a three-dimensional object often it is difficult to assess the degree and extent of bone loss based on the radiographs. Clinical examination also helps to evaluate trauma from occlusion, tooth mobility, open contacts, and local irritating factors such as smoking, mouth breathing, crowding of teeth, plaque, and calculus.

LIMITATIONS OF RADIOGRAPHS

- Radiographs cannot be used in the diagnosis of even severe infections confined to the gingiva
- Initial bone changes may not be apparent in the radiograph
- Superimposition of buccal and lingual bone makes it difficult to determine the bone loss
- The dense image of the roots superimposed obscures the height of the bone
- Soft tissue and hard tissue relationship cannot be determined
- Radiographically it may not be possible to differentiate between a diseased state and successfully treated case
- The actual extent of bone destruction may be more than what is visualized in the radiograph.

The ideal radiograph to study the periodontal disease is a properly taken bitewing radiograph. An important factor helping in the diagnosis of periodontal disease is the radiographic relationship of cementoenamel junction (CEJ) with the crest of the alveolus. Normally the distance between the CEJ and crest of the alveolus is 1–1.5 mm. This distance is altered in periodontal disease due to the destruction of alveolar bone.

RADIOGRAPHIC FEATURES OF PERIODONTAL DISEASE

Based on the clinical stage and the radiographic features, the periodontal disease (periodontitis) may be classified into three types:
- Early periodontitis
- Moderate periodontitis
- Advanced periodontitis.

EARLY PERIODONTITIS

Early periodontitis is associated with minimal bone changes. This stage is characterized by loss of sharp edge of the alveolar crest as seen in the radiograph of anterior region (Fig. 16-1).

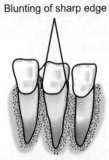

Fig. 16-1: Bone loss in the anterior region

In the posterior region there may be blunting of the sharp angle formed by the lamina dura and the alveolar crest (Fig. 16-2).

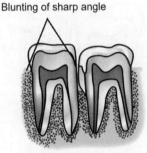

Fig. 16-2: Bone loss in the region posterior region

In some radiographs, an artefact of severe bone loss may be evident due to variation in the angulation of the radiographic projection.

MODERATE PERIODONTITIS

In moderate periodontitis, the alveolar bone destruction has progressed. It is often associated with bony defects. There may also be loss of cortical plates. Defects of the bone are usually seen in the interradicular or the interdental bone between the buccal and the lingual cortical plates. There can also be localized or generalized horizontal bone loss.

The following radiographic changes are seen associated with moderate periodontitis.

i. Horizontal bone loss

ii. Osseous defects
- Interproximal crater
- Proximal intrabony defect
- Interproximal hemisepta
- Inconsistent bony margins
- Bony pockets.

(i) Horizontal Bone Loss

Horizontal bone loss is characterized by reduction in the height of the alveolar bone in a horizontal direction (Fig. 16-3). It may be localized or generalized based on the regions involved.

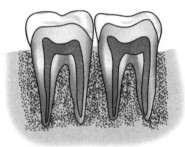

Fig. 16-3: Horizontal bone loss

It can also be mild, moderate, or severe based on the extent of bone loss. The horizontal bone loss usually involves the buccal and the lingual cortical plates and the interdental bone.

(ii) Osseous Defects

The term osseous defects is generalized to describe all bony changes associated with periodontal disease, other than the horizontal bone loss.

Interproximal Crater

Interproximal crater is a trough-like or saucer-shaped defect occurring in the alveolar crest of the interproximal bone. The bony defect has four walls: the buccal and lingual cortical plates and the roots of two adjacent teeth. The marginal bone of the interproximal crater appears thin.

Proximal Intrabony Defect

Proximal intrabony defect is a vertical defect of bone, extending from the crest of the alveolus and in an apical direction. It is a defect surrounded by four walls; the buccal and the lingual cortical plates, the hemiseptum, and the root of the involved tooth. Radiographically the proximal intrabony defect appears 'V'-shaped, adjacent to the affected root surface.

Interproximal Hemisepta

A hemiseptum is defined as the bone of the interdental septum that remains on the root of the uninvolved adjacent tooth after destruction of either the mesial or the distal portion of the interproximal bone septum. The hemiseptum results due to the loss of bone on the mesial or the distal aspect of a root surface. Radiographically, the hemiseptum is 'V' or 'U'-shaped, (Fig. 16-4).

Inconsistent Bony Margins

Inconsistent bony margins refer to irregular resorption of the cortical bone of the buccal or lingual alveolar cortical plate. Radiographically this bony change appears as irregular loss of the height of the alveolar crest.

Hemiseptum

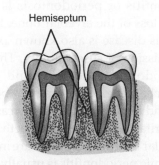

Fig. 16-4: Hemiseptum

Bony Pockets

Bony pockets usually occur together with proximal bony defects. Bony pockets are seen on the buccal aspect of the roots. Radiographs may not be very useful in the diagnosis of bony defects on the buccal or the lingual cortex.

ADVANCED PERIODONTITIS

Advanced periodontitis is clinically characterized by mobility of the involved teeth. Radiographically there will be extensive horizontal bone loss or osseous defects.

Defects in Furcation Area

Bony defects are seen in the furcation area of multirooted teeth. Bone loss in the furcation area is manifested radiographically as radiolucency in the involved region. Furcation involvement may not be readily visualized in the maxillary radiographs because of the superimposition of the palatal root.

Alveolar Dehiscence

Alveolar dehiscence refers to the apical dipping of the marginal alveolar bone. It can occur either on the buccal side or on the lingual side. The level of bone is apparent as a radiopaque line with faint image of the trabeculae.

JUVENILE PERIODONTITIS

Juvenile periodontitis or periodontosis is characterized by severe and rapid loss of the alveolar bone. Familial pattern of distribution of this disease is also known, possibly as a result of genetic transmission of susceptibility. There are two forms of juvenile periodontitis: localized and generalized. The localized form is characterized by angular bone loss involving the first molars and the incisors. In many cases there is virtual absence of local irritants. The maxillary teeth are involved more than the mandibular teeth and the teeth are involved bilaterally. The onset of juvenile periodontitis is usually after adolescence. Many of the affected individuals have an inherited defect of neutrophil chemotactic function.

In the generalized form there is involvement of many teeth. It usually has a late onset, usually occurring between 20 and 30 years of age. Apart from the first molars and the incisors, the generalized form involves the canines, the premolars, and the second molars. It is also considered as an extension of the local form, whereas others believe that it is a type of rapidly progressive periodontitis.

Chapter 17

Radiographic Features of Traumatic Injuries: Fracture of the Teeth and Jaws

- *Introduction*
- *Traumatic Injuries Involving the Teeth*
- *Traumatic Injuries Involving the Jaws*
- *Radiographic Features of Fracture of the Jaws*
  Fracture of mandible
  Classification of fractures
  Fracture of maxillofacial complex
  Radiographic features of fractures of maxilla
  Zygomatic fractures

You, to whom your Maker granted
Powers to those sweet birds unknown,
  Use the craft by God implanted;
Use the reason not your own.
  Here, while heaven and earth rejoices,
Each his Easter tribute bring-
  Work of fingers, chant of voices,
Like the birds who build and sing.

– **Charles Kingsley**

INTRODUCTION

Trauma can be defined as an injury produced by an external force. Traumatic injuries can involve the teeth alone, the jaws alone or the teeth and the jaws. The degree and extent of the injuries depend on the severity of the trauma. Though intraoral films suffice in the diagnosis of traumatic injuries involving the teeth, extraoral radiographs are required in the evaluation of traumatic injuries to the jaws.

TRAUMATIC INJURIES INVOLVING THE TEETH

Traumatic injuries to the teeth can cause various injuries such as concussion, luxation (intrusive, extrusive and lateral), avulsion or fractures.

Concussion

In concussion there is crushing injury to the apical vasculature and the periodontal ligament of the apical region leading to inflammatory edema. Thus, concussion is essentially an injury to the supporting tissues of the teeth.

The patient reports pain. As there is accumulation of inflammatory edema in the apical region, the involved tooth may be slightly elevated from the socket. This results in pain while biting. The radiographic change that is noticeable in concussion is widening of the periodontal ligament space at the apex. Evidence of pulpal necrosis and periapical lesion may be noted after a variable period of time.

Luxation

Luxation of the teeth refers to dislocation or loosening of the teeth due to loss of the periodontal attachment. The loosening can be:

- **Intrusive luxation:** Intrusive luxation results when the tooth is displaced into the alveolar bone
- **Extrusive luxation:** Extrusive luxation refers to displacement of the tooth out of the socket
- **Lateral luxation:** In lateral luxation, the tooth is displaced to the side.

In majority of the cases luxation involves the anterior teeth. The clinical features are the following:

- The affected tooth may be mobile
- Bleeding through the gingival crevice
- Tenderness on percussion.

In intrusive luxation the tooth will be pushed into the socket and the crown length appears shortened compared to the adjacent teeth. In extrusive luxation the tooth will be pushed out of the socket and the crown appears elongated.

The radiographic changes seen may be variable. In intrusive luxation there is disruption of the continuity of the lamina dura in the apical region, whereas in extrusive luxation there is widening of the periodontal ligament space in the periapical region which is radiographically apparent as periapical radiolucency. In case of lateral luxation there is widening of the periodontal ligament space on one side and obliteration of the periodontal ligament space on the other side with evidence of damage to the lamina dura of the involved side. Either pulpal necrosis or calcification of the pulp chamber and the root canal can occur eventually which will be radiographically evident as periapical lesion or obliteration of the pulp chamber and the root canal.

Avulsion

Avulsion or exarticulation refers to complete displacement of the tooth from its socket. Often the teeth involved are the maxillary incisors. Clinically the tooth will be absent and the socket appears empty, except for blood or blood clot. The radiographic appearance of avulsion is an empty socket. The radiographic examination can also be used to rule out displacement of the tooth into the adjacent soft tissues.

Fracture of the Teeth

Fracture of a tooth is defined as the breaking of tooth parts. The maxillary incisors are more prone for fracture especially in those individuals with proclined anterior teeth. The children are more prone for traumatic injuries. Accordingly, the deciduous teeth have a slightly greater affliction.

Coronal fractures of teeth can be broadly classified into the following three groups.

  i. Fractures involving only the enamel and without any loss of tooth structure (infarction or crack)

ii. Fracture involving the enamel or the enamel and the dentin with loss of tooth structure and without involvement of the pulp (uncomplicated fracture)

iii. Fractures involving the enamel, the dentin, and the pulp with loss of tooth structure (complicated fracture)

Bennett's Classification of Fracture of Teeth

The Bennett's classification can be used in the evaluation of coronal and root fracture. In this classification, the injured tooth is classified into five classes (Table 17-1).

Table 17-1: Bennett's classification of fracture of teeth

Class I	Traumatized tooth without coronal or root fracture
	A. Tooth firm in alveolus
	B. Tooth subluxed in alveolus
Class II	Coronal fracture
	A. Involving enamel
	B. Involving enamel and dentin
Class III	Coronal fracture with pulpal exposure
Class IV	Root fracture
	A. Without coronal fracture
	B. With coronal fracture
Class V	Avulsion of tooth

Various clinical features of fractures of the teeth are crack on the enamel surface; loss of the enamel usually on the mesial or distal side, or loss of tooth structure on the incisal edge; loss of tooth structure involving the enamel and the dentin with or without pulp exposure; and mobility of crown when there is root fracture (Fig. 17-1). If there is pulpal exposure, the pulp

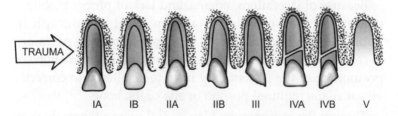

Fig. 17-1: Diagrammatic representation of various traumatic injuries of the teeth

tissue will be clinically visible as a reddish tiny mass. Exposed dentin, in case of fractures involving the enamel and the dentin will be sensitive to mechanical and thermal stimulation. The root fracture of the anterior teeth usually occurs in the midportion of the teeth resulting in mobility of the crown. In case of complicated fractures there is loss of tooth parts.

The radiographic features of fracture of the teeth are
- Radiolucent line between tooth segments
- Displacement of tooth fragments
- Disruption of the continuity of the tooth surface
- In case of root fracture, there may be a radiolucent line traversing the midportion of the tooth suggestive of fracture
- Oblique fracture line may be mistaken as two fracture lines as radiographically the radiolucent lines may be evident separately in two planes.

TRAUMATIC INJURIES INVOLVING THE JAWS

Radiographic Features of Fracture of the Jaws

The traumatic injuries to the jaws and the other facial bones are mainly due to road traffic accidents, fall, and assault. It goes without saying that a thorough knowledge of the anatomy of the facial bones and their radiographic appearance is absolutely essential in the diagnosis of fractures. The clinician should also know which radiographs to ask for in the evaluation of maxillofacial trauma.

Because of lacerations, edema, and lack of proper mobility, it may not be possible to take an ideal radiograph in traumatized patients. Multiple radiographs may be necessary to confirm or rule out a fracture. Sometimes the angulations or positioning of the patient may have to be altered to correctly visualize the required portion or site of the bone.

Though the radiographs play a vital role in the evaluation of mandibular and maxillofacial trauma, the importance of clinical examination cannot be overruled.

Radiographic Features of Fractures

The various radiographic features of fractures are:
  i. Demonstration of fracture line which radiographically appears as a radiolucent line.
 ii. Displacement of adjacent bony segments. Often displacement cannot be identified in a single radiographic projection. Multiple radiographs, probably at right angles to each other may be required.
iii. Alteration of bony contour. Fractures and displacement result in alteration of the bony shape, the size, and the contour. This is very important in the diagnosis of fracture.

Fracture of Mandible

The main radiographic projections made in the diagnosis of fracture of the mandible are:
- Orthopantomogram (OPG)
- Lateral oblique view
- Posteroanterior (PA) or anteroposterior (AP) view
- Reverse Towne view (for condyles, condylar neck, and rami).

Sometimes additional TMJ views are required in the diagnosis of fractures involving the condyle or coronoid process.

Classification of Fractures

A fracture can be classified into three types.
  A. **Greenstick fracture:** In the Greenstick fracture, only one side of the cortex is broken or the fracture is present in one cortex of the bone and the opposite side is bent.
  B. **Simple fracture:** In case of simple fracture, there is no communication of the fracture to the external environment.
  C. **Compound fracture:** In compound fracture, the fracture is exposed to external environment, either the skin surface or mucous membrane.

A fracture of the mandible can occur at different sites. These sites are the symphysis, the parasymphysis, the body, the angle, the ramus, the alveolar process, the condylar process, and the coronoid process (Fig. 17-2).

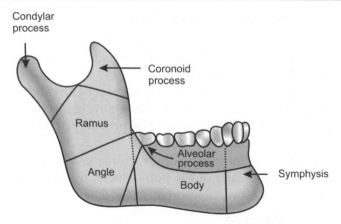

Fig. 17-2: Different sites of mandibular fractures

Condylar fractures may be either intraarticular (intracapsular) or subcondylar (extracapsular). Intraarticular fractures are relatively rare compared to extraarticular fractures. Subcondylar fractures occur between the condylar head and the junction of the condylar neck with the ramus of the mandible. In most of the cases of fracture of the condyle, the condyle gets displaced anteriorly and medially due to the action of the lateral pterygoid muscle. In the radiographs, the condylar fractures can be identified based on the alteration of the shape of the condyle due to this displacement.

Fracture of the coronoid process of the mandible is extremely rare as it is well-protected by the zygomatic arch. But severely depressed zygomatic arch fracture can result in the fracture of the coronoid process. Coronoid fracture is best visualized in lateral oblique view.

As the mandibular ramus is composed of dense bone, fracture of the ramus is very rare. Fracture of the ramus occurs due to direct trauma to the ramus.

The angle of the mandible is susceptible for fracture because of the alteration in the trabecular pattern and the impacted third molars contributing to weakening of this site. If the fracture line extends obliquely from anterior to posterior direction, the ramus can get displaced superolaterally due to the action of the muscle attachment in this region. Hence, this type of fracture is termed unfavorable fracture. If the fracture line extends in a superoposterior to an inferoanterior direction, the proximal fragment gets locked below the distal fragment and thus resisting the action of the muscles (masseter and internal pterygoid). This type of fracture is termed as a favorable fracture.

The fracture of the mandible can occur in the symphysis, the mental, the submental, the cuspid, and the molar regions. Another way of classifying the mandibular body fracture is to group them into the symphysis or the midline fractures, the para symphysis fractures, and the body fractures. Fracture of the mandible is evidenced as radiolucent line or step-like deformity. Displacement of the fractured fragments should be identified based on occlusal projection. Bilateral fractures of body of the mandible can cause inferior displacement and deformation of the anterior segment due to the action of the suprahyoid muscle. There can be displacement in obliquely directed fracture of the symphysis.

Fractures involving the symphysis and the parasymphysis are rare and on many occasions occur in association with fractures at other sites.

Fracture of the alveolar process usually occurs on the buccal surface. Orthopantomogram is a good projection to visualize horizontal alveolar fracture.

The common traumatic injuries involving the TMJ are subluxation and dislocation. In subluxation the head of the condyle lies in a position anterior and superior to the articular eminence and the patient can reduce the condyle to its original position without any professional manipulation. Dislocation is similar to subluxation, but the patient cannot reduce the mandible.

Dislocation of the TMJ occurs due to blow to the mandible and is often bilateral. Dislocation can also occur due to TMJ dysfunction and muscular incoordination. The dislocated mandible can be repositioned by downward and posterior pressure, keeping the fingers on the buccal surface of the posterior teeth. Diazepam is often helpful in calming the patient and in relaxing the muscles.

In certain rare situations, the mandibular condyle may get dislocated into the middle cranial cavity through the glenoid fossa (cranial dislocation). The clinical features of cranial dislocation are limitation of mandibular movement and premature occlusal contact of the affected side.

If the condylar fracture is unilateral, the contralateral body of the mandible may be fractured, whereas if the condylar fracture is bilateral, the additional fracture line may be seen in the symphysis region.

Healing of fracture of the condyle occurs in a rotated or tilted position and the condyle appears deformed. The inferior segment may become the new articular surface.

In the orthopantomogram and lateral oblique view, the palatolingual and the palatopharyngeal airspaces superimposed over the mandible may be mistaken for fracture lines. Superimposition of the hyoid bone, the intervertebral spaces in the symphyseal region, and the elongated styloid process can also be erroneously mistaken for fracture. The nutrient canals in the anterior region also should not be mistaken for fracture, especially in the edentulous patients.

Fractures of the Maxillofacial Complex

The diagnosis of the maxillofacial complex fractures is very difficult due to the superimposition of several anatomic structures with the result that the facial radiographs appear very complex. Various radiographic projections that can be used in the evaluation of the maxillofacial trauma are lateral jaw projection, Waters view, submentovertex view, and maxillary occlusal radiograph.

The evaluation of four "S" is very useful in correct radiographic interpretation.
- Symmetry
- Sharpness

- Sinus
- Soft tissues.

The symmetry should be checked in cases of fractures of the zygoma, the nose, the maxillary sinus, and the orbit. The term sharpness is used with reference to the margins of bones or bone fragments. The different radiographic signs used to describe facial injuries are 'trap door' (due to fracture of the orbital floor), 'bright-light' (due to free bone fragment within the maxillary sinus), and 'railroad track' (due to an additional fracture line on the lateral aspect of the orbit because of tripod fracture and rotation of the zygoma). The radiographic signs of the sinus trauma are haziness of the sinus due to edema, well-defined mass due to herniation of the orbital contents, generalized opacification or fluid level due to intraluminal bleeding secondary to a mucosal tear, or loss of integrity of the bony outline. In case of blow-out fractures there can be soft tissue mass due to submucosal and intramucosal herniation.

Depending on the location of the injury, the maxillofacial trauma may warrant three to five films. These views are Waters, Caldwell, and lateral views. The additional views required are the submentovertex view (for the zygomatic arch), reverse Towne, and nasal views.

The Waters and Caldwell views are very useful in the evaluation of trauma. The Waters view visualizes the maxillary sinus and the anterior facial structures, whereas the Caldwell view visualizes the orbits and the posterior facial structures.

There are three lines used in the evaluation of trauma, to the zygoma, the orbit, and the nose. These are the maxillary, the zygomatic, and the orbital lines. The maxillary line runs along the outline of the lateral wall of the maxillary sinus and the undersurface of the zygomatic arch. The zygomatic line runs along the lateral and the superior surface of the zygoma and the zygomatic arch from the zygomatic process of the frontal bone to the TMJ. These two lines help in the evaluation of zygomatic trauma. The orbital line extends from the nasion along the infraorbital rim to the zygomatic process of the frontal bone. This line is useful in the evaluation of the orbital, the Le Fort II, and the nasoethmoid midfacial fractures.

Alternately the maxillofacial area can be divided into four areas with the help of four curvilinear lines described by McGrigor and Campbell (1950) (Fig. 17-3).

1. The first line starts from the zygomaticofrontal suture of one side along the supraorbital margin and across the glabella to the supraorbital margin and the zygomaticofrontal suture of the opposite side.

2. The second line extends from superior aspect of the zygomatic arch and the zygoma to the zygomaticofrontal suture, along the infraorbital margin, across the frontal process of the maxilla, along the lateral wall of the nose, through the nasal septum, and then proceeding in the same manner to the opposite side.

3. The third line extends from the mandibular condyles across the sigmoid notch and the tip of the coronoid process to

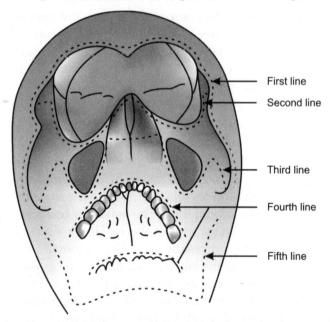

Fig. 17-3: McGrigor and Campbell lines

the lateral and medial antral walls at the level of the nasal floor and having a similar course in the opposite side.

4. The fourth line runs across the occlusal plane of the upper and the lower teeth. If the patient is edentulous, the line extends through the crest of the alveolar ridge.

A fifth line is also described extending through the lower border of the mandible and the posterior aspect of the ramus.

The intervertebral spaces seen in the posteroanterior projection may be mistaken for the fracture of the alveolar process or a Le Fort I fracture of the maxilla.

Radiographic Features of Fractures of Maxilla

Fractures of the maxilla can involve the alveolar process, the body of the maxilla, and the maxilla with adjacent facial bones. Fracture can also occur as a part in craniofacial dysjunction. In blow-out fractures of the floor of the orbit there is involvement of superior maxillary antral wall without involvement of the maxilla.

The sites of maxillary fractures can be grouped as given below:

- Fracture of the alveolus
- Horizontal maxillary fracture (Le Fort I)
- Pyramidal maxillary fracture (Le Fort II)
- Craniofacial dysjunction (Le Fort III)
- Blow-out fracture of the orbit.

The alveolar process fracture is identifiable in the periapical radiographs as regular or irregular radiolucent line. Sometimes prominent nutrient canals may be mistaken for fracture.

In Le Fort I fracture, the fracture line passes above the teeth, below the zygomatic process, through the maxillary sinuses, the tuberosities to the inferior portion of the pterygoid processes. In Le Fort I fracture, the maxillary tooth-bearing segment is detached from the middle face.

In some cases, the horizontal maxillary fractures may be unilateral, that involves the lateral wall of the antrum, along with the pterygoid plates on one side and the midpalatal suture. Maxillary occlusal projection is very useful in determining the palatal fracture line.

In Le Fort II or pyramidal fractures, the fracture line extends laterally through the lacrimal bones, floors of the orbit, and inferiorly through the zygomaticomaxillary sutures. Often on one side the fracture passes through the suture or through the zygoma and on the other side it passes around and beneath the base of the zygomatic process of the maxilla. In the posteroanterior view Le Fort II fracture appears pyramidal. Hence the name pyramidal fracture for this type of fracture. The Le Fort II fracture is characterized by edema, and circumorbital ecchymosis. If the zygomatic bones are involved there can be subconjunctival ecchymosis.

In Le Fort III fracture or craniofacial dysjunction, the fracture line extends through the nasal bones and the frontal process of the maxillae or the nasofrontal and the maxillofrontal sutures, across the orbits, through the ethmoid and the sphenoid sinuses and the zygomaticofrontal sutures. There is separation of the pterygoid plates and the maxillae are displaced and movable. In Le Fort III fractures, the soft tissue injuries are severe. There is severe edema and cerebrospinal fluid (CSF) rhinorrhea. The face will have 'dish face" appearance and anterior open bite.

The orbital floor fracture occurs due to sufficient force applied in the ocular region. As the inferior orbital floor is weak, the force causes downward rupture of this bony plate into the maxillary antrum. There can be herniation of the orbital contents such as fat and a portion of inferior rectus muscle. Waters projection is very ideal in the evaluation of the orbital floor fracture. Hemorrhage into the maxillary sinus may obscure a blow-out fracture.

Zygomatic Fractures

The zygoma is a prominent bone in the facial structure. It acts as a bridge between the lower face and calvarium. It has a central body and four processes (the frontal, the temporal, the maxillary, and the infraorbital). Through the sutural attachments it articulates with five bones (the zygomatic process of the frontal and the temporal bones, the medial maxilla at the orbital rim, the maxillary alveolus, and the sphenoid bone in the anterolateral orbit). The fractures of the zygoma are divided into the tripod fracture and the isolated zygomatic fracture.

In tripod fracture there is involvement of the malar, the zygomaticomaxillary and the zygomatic complex. The tripod fracture results from a horizontally directed blow to the zygoma or the zygomatic arch, resulting in disruption of the three major attachments. The disruptions are at the zygomaticotemporal, the zygomaticomaxillary and the zygomaticofrontal articulations. The various radiographic projections used in the evaluation of tripod fractures are Waters, Caldwell, submentovertex and Towne views.

The Waters view visualizes the zygomatic arch, the lateral wall of the maxillary sinus, the infraorbital rim and the floor of the orbit. Caldwell projection is useful in the evaluation of the frontal process of the zygoma and the lateral orbit in cases of fractures involving the zygomaticofrontal suture and the lateral orbit. The submentovertex view helps in the evaluation of fracture of the zygomatic arch. Towne view is helpful to determine the lateral or the medial rotation of the zygoma.

The zygomatic arch is made up of the zygomatic process of the temporal bone and the temporal process of the zygoma. These fractures result due to a horizontally directed force striking the temporal process of the zygoma posterior to the body of the zygoma. The injuries range from mild bowing to comminuted depressed fractures of the zygomatic arch that involves both the temporal and the zygomatic components. Sometimes fracture of the proximal end can extend to involve the glenoid fossa.

The zygomatic arch fracture may be determined based on submentovertex view and Waters view. The radiographic signs are:

- Depression of the zygomatic arch
- Vertical radiopaque band lateral to the body of the zygoma
- 'W'-shaped deformity due to fracture of the temporal process of the zygoma and zygomatic process of the temporal bone
- Diastasis of the zygomaticofrontal suture.

Chapter 18

Inflammation and Infections of the Jaws

- *Introduction*
- *Infections of the Supporting Tissues of the Teeth*
- *Pericoronitis and Pericoronal Infection*
- *Periapical and Residual Infections*
- *Osteomyelitis*
- *Actinomycosis*
- *Cellulitis*
- *Ludwig's Angina*

The wind blows out, the bubble dies;
The spring entombed in autumn lies;
The dew dries up, the star is shot;
The flight is past, and man forgot.

– Henry King, Bishop of Chichester

INTRODUCTION

The vast majority of infections involving the jaws are nonspecific bacterial infections and most of them are dental in origin. The infections of the jaws can be grouped under:

- i. Infections of the supporting tissues of the teeth (e.g. periodontal diseases)
- ii. Pericoronitis and pericoronal infection
- iii. Periapical and residual infections
- iv. Osteomyelitis
- v. Actinomycosis

vi. Cellulitis

vii. Ludwig's Angina

INFECTIONS OF THE SUPPORTING TISSUES OF THE TEETH

The supporting tissues of the teeth are the gingiva, the periodontal ligament, the alveolar bone, and the cementum. The inflammation and infection of the supporting tissues originate in the soft tissue component of the periodontium, that is, the gingiva and later on progressing to involve the supporting alveolar bone. When there is destruction of the alveolar bone there will be radiographic evidence of periodontal disease. The radiographic features of periodontal diseases are discussed in detail in Chapter 16.

PERICORONITIS AND PERICORONAL INFECTION

Pericoronitis is a term given for inflammation surrounding the soft tissues of the teeth, usually the erupting third molars. Prolonged soft tissue infection can progress to cause destruction of the adjacent alveolar bone. Acute and chronic abscess occurs in association with partially erupted or impacted teeth. The most frequently involved teeth are the mandibular third molars. The clinical findings are pain and inflammatory changes of the pericoronal flap. There may also be swelling and pus discharge on digital pressure as infection sets in. There can also be considerable bleeding on probing the affected area. Clinically, food enlodgement and deep pocket may be readily visible. Radiographic examination reveals crater-like bony defect in the retromolar region.

PERIAPICAL AND RESIDUAL INFECTIONS

The periapical infection is usually a sequela of necrosis of the pulp. This can also result from blood-borne microorganisms. The main causes of pulpal necrosis are:

• Caries
• Improper restoration with defective margins
• Defective base

- Incomplete removal of the caries before placement of the restoration
- Secondary caries
- Cavity preparation without coolants
- Fracture of the teeth
- Spread of infection through the periodontal ligament space.

Acute Periapical Abscess

Acute periapical infection is the result of infection from the tooth reaching the periapical region, where it causes destruction of the surrounding bone. The initial radiographic change is widening of the periodontal ligament space, subsequently producing more extensive destruction of the supporting alveolar bone in the periapical region. The acute periapical abscess can become a chronic abscess or a periapical granuloma.

Chronic Periapical Abscess

When the acute phase of a periapical infection subsides, the chronic phase ensues characterized by less severe symptoms. Pain and swelling are variable features. Sometimes an intraoral sinus is noted through which pus and serum are released. In some cases the sinus may open to the surface of the skin extraorally. The radiographic appearance is diffuse radiolucency involving the affected tooth in the periapical region.

Periapical Granuloma

Periapical granuloma is a reparative process occurring in case of periapical abscess. A periapical granuloma can also result from spread of infection from the periodontal ligament space into the periapical region. Histologically, the periapical granuloma contains lymphocytes and plasma cells. Radiographically, it appears as a round or oval radiolucency in the periapical region of the involved tooth. The radiolucency is less than 1 cm in diameter and surrounded by a well-defined sclerotic border. In some cases there can be resorption of the root in the apical region.

Residual Infection

The term residual infection refers to the persistence of infection even after the extraction of the involved tooth. In many cases there is presence of retained root stumps which act as the source of infection. The residual infection can also result from a tooth affected by chronic periapical abscess, even after the extraction of the affected tooth. Radiographically it appears as an area of radiolucency with diffuse borders. Sometimes retained root stumps may be evident in the radiograph.

OSTEOMYELITIS

The term osteomyelitis refers to inflammation of the bone (Fig. 18-1). In majority of the cases the origin or source of infection is from periapical infections, periodontal diseases, pericoronitis, trauma to the jaws, infection of the maxillary sinus, chronic local infections of the face, postirradiation period, and any infection of the socket after the tooth extraction. Some of the systemic infections that can cause osteomyelitis are syphilis, tuberculosis, and actinomycosis.

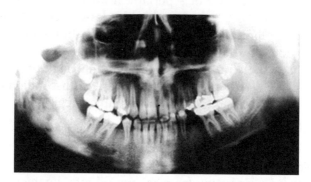

Fig. 18-1: Osteomyelitis as visualized in panoramic radiograph

Acute Osteomyelitis

Acute osteomyelitis is characterized by sudden onset of pain, elevation of temperature, pus discharge, mobility of the involved teeth and ultimately leading to necrosis of the bone and formation of sequestrum.

In the initial phase of the infection, radiographic changes may not be evident. The initial radiographic changes are destruction of the bone, visualized as irregular areas of radiolucency. The dead bone or sequestrum may also be evident radiographically as detached fragments of bone.

The management involves initiation of antibiotic therapy, drainage, or extraction of the offending teeth.

Diffuse Sclerosing Osteomyelitis

Chronic diffuse sclerosing osteomyelitis is a proliferative reaction of the bone to a low-grade infection. This is usually seen in elderly individuals. The radiographic features are obliteration of the marrow spaces and thickening of the cortical plates. There may also be enlargement of the bone as evidenced in occlusal radiograph. Radiographic appearance of this lesion may be similar to that of Paget's disease of bone.

Infantile Osteomyelitis

Infantile osteomyelitis or hematogenous osteomyelitis occurs in children and adolescents, usually as a sequela of systemic infections such as measles, scarlet fever, and skin infections. There can be involvement of many bones. The radiographic appearance of the lesion is a diffuse radiolucency.

Garré's Osteomyelitis (Periostitis ossificans)

In Garré's osteomyelitis, the infection is localized in the periosteum and produces expansion of the bone on the outer surface of the cortex (subperiosteal deposition of bone). It usually occurs in children and young adults, in the mandible. The characteristic radiographic appearance is onion-skin appearance. The other lesions to be considered in the differential diagnosis are Caffey's disease (infantile cortical hyperostosis), Ewing's sarcoma, osteogenic sarcoma and fracture callus.

ACTINOMYCOSIS

Actinomycosis is a specific bacterial infection caused by *Actinomyces israelii*. The infection is characterized by granulomatous changes with multiple sinuses through which yellow granules (sulfur granules) are released. The cervicofacial actinomycosis is associated with swelling, trismus, pain and fever. The infection can originate from contaminated extraction socket, periodontal pocket, or infected and necrosed pulp tissue. The mandible is the favored site. The radiographic findings are variable, either appearing as a periapical granuloma or as diffuse areas of bone destruction.

CELLULITIS

Cellulitis is the inflammation of the soft tissues due to tracking of pus through tissue spaces and facial planes. It usually follows a periapical abscess, osteomyelitis or pericoronitis. The features of cellulitis are painful swelling, stretching of the skin surface with redness, fever, leukocytosis, and lymphadenitis. Radiographic finding is diffuse radiolucency in the periapical region of the involved tooth.

LUDWIG'S ANGINA

Ludwig's angina is a severe form of cellulitis with involvement of the submaxillary, the sublingual and the submental spaces. The infection may originate from the infected mandibular molars. The thin lingual plate facilitates the spread of infection to the floor of the mouth. From this region the infection spreads to the neck. In some cases there can be edema of the glottis. The radiographic changes are seen at the periapical region of the involved tooth and are similar to that of periapical infection.

Cysts of the Jaws

An opal-hearted country,
A wilful, lavish land ......
All who have not loved her,
You will not understand ......
Though earth holds many splendors,
Wherever I may die,
I know to what brown country
My homing thoughts will fly.

— **Dorothea Mackellar**

INTRODUCTION

A cyst is an epithelium-lined cavity, containing gaseous, semisolid, or fluid material, but not pus. The cysts of the jaws may be divided into odontogenic and nonodontogenic cysts. The cysts have a tendency to expand due to the tension as a result of an osmotic imbalance. The cysts assume a globular pattern because of the expansion in all directions (Fig. 19-1).

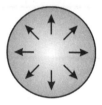

Fig. 19-1: Expansion of a cyst

ODONTOGENIC CYSTS

Radicular Cyst

A radicular cyst is also called as periapical cyst. It occurs as a sequela of periapical infection resulting from caries or traumatic injuries to the teeth (Fig. 19-2).

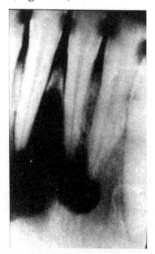

Fig. 19-2: Periapical cyst

The origin of a cyst may be from the lining of the granulation tissue in the periapical region epithelial and further cystic degeneration of the inner mass of cells which becomes devoid of nutritional supply and undergoes liquefaction necrosis.

The periapical cyst is lined with squamous epithelium. Radiographically periapical cyst appears as a large round radiolucency, greater than 1 cm in diameter with a sclerotic border. If the cyst becomes infected, the border becomes less distinct.

Other lesions to be considered in the differential diagnosis of periapical cyst are periapical granuloma, periapical scar and surgical defect.

Dentigerous Cyst

Dentigerous cyst is also called as follicular cyst or pericoronal cyst. The dentigerous cyst originates due to the cystic changes occurring in an enamel organ after the crown has been formed. It usually occurs in association with the crowns of unerupted teeth. The teeth usually involved are the mandibular third molars, the maxillary canines and the premolars. A dentigerous cyst can also occur in association with the supernumerary teeth.

Most of the dentigerous cysts are solitary. Bilateral cysts occur in association with basal cell nevus bifid rib syndrome and cleidocranial dysplasia. About 10% of all dentigerous cysts are odontogenic keratocysts.

Radiographically the dentigerous cyst appears as a well-defined radiolucency with a sclerotic or hyperostotic border in association with the crown of an unerupted tooth. Usually the cyst is unilocular. However, rarely it exhibits a multilocular pattern.

Various lesions to be considered in the differential diagnosis are ameloblastoma, calcifying epithelial odontogenic cyst, ameloblastic fibroma or adenomatoid odontogenic tumor.

Residual Cyst

Residual cysts must have remained or developed after extraction of teeth, from the residual epithelial rests. The residual cysts are usually seen in patients over the age of 20 years. The residual cyst can occur anywhere in the jaws. Many cases are asymptomatic, discovered only during routine radiographic examination. Radiographic examination reveals round or ovoid radiolucency with sclerotic border. The hyperostotic border may be lost due to infection.

The lesions to be considered in the differential diagnosis are primordial cyst, odontogenic keratocyst and traumatic bone cyst.

Odontogenic Keratocyst

Odontogenic keratocyst is characterized by keratinization of its epithelial lining. This cyst accounts for 11% of all jaw cysts. The incidence of odontogenic keratocyst is highest in the second and the third decades and it has more male predilection. The odontogenic keratocysts more predominantly occur in the mandible, in the angle region and extending into the ramus. Cases have also been reported in the globulomaxillary area. Pain is a symptom only if the cyst is infected. Expansion of the cyst is rather slow.

The typical radiographic appearance of an odontogenic keratocyst is a multilocular radiolucency with undulating borders and cloudy interior. The borders are hyperostotic. There may be displacement of the teeth. The maxillary lesions are usually smaller and unilocular.

Calcifying Odontogenic Cyst

Calcifying odontogenic cyst is characterized by calcification of the walls of the lesion. It occurs more predominantly in the mandible than in the maxilla. The age of occurrence may vary from 8–74 years and there is no sex predilection.

Radiographically it appears as a unilocular cystic space. Scattered radiopaque spots are present at the borders and also within the radiolucent area.

As the cyst walls are thicker, the cyst can be enucleated easily.

Primordial Cyst

Primordial cyst originates due to cystic changes occurring within the stellate reticulum of a tooth germ before the initiation of mineralization. Thus, it occurs in the place of a tooth. Rarely it can also occur in the place of a supernumerary tooth. It predominantly affects children and young adults. It can also attain a large size. It has a high recurrence rate.

Radiographically it appears as a unilocular or multilocular lesion. The outline may be scalloped. It may mimic a dentigerous cyst. There can be displacement of the adjacent teeth. Rarely lesions have been reported in the globulomaxillary area. One school of thought believes that the globulomaxillary cyst is not a fissural cyst, but is a primordial cyst occurring in the place of a supernumerary tooth.

Various lesions to be considered in the differential diagnosis are odontogenic keratocyst, residual cyst, traumatic bone cyst, early ameloblastoma and myxoma.

Globulomaxillary Cyst

Currently, the globulomaxillary cyst is considered to be odontogenic in origin. These cysts occur in the globulomaxillary region and are usually detected during routine radiographic examination. They can cause expansion of the cortical plate. There can also be divergence of the roots of lateral incisor and canine.

Radiographically it appears as a pear-shaped or tear-shaped radiolucency between the roots of the lateral incisor and the canine. The narrow end of the cyst is directed downward to the alveolar crest.

In the differential diagnosis, lateral fossa, dentigerous cyst, adenomatoid odontogenic tumor or surgical defect should be considered.

Median Mandibular Cyst

Median mandibular cyst is a rare cyst occurring in the region of the symphysis. Its origin is debatable. It may originate as a primordial cyst of a supernumerary tooth, lateral periodontal cyst or a radicular cyst. Radiographically it is round or ovoid with regular or diffuse borders.

NONODONTOGENIC CYSTS

Incisive Canal Cyst or Nasopalatine Cyst

Incisive canal cyst is also called as median anterior maxillary cyst. It is the most common nonodontogenic cyst occurring in the maxilla. It originates due to the cystic transformation of the epithelial remnants of the nasopalatine duct. This cyst is usually discovered in the fourth to sixth decades of life.

Radiographically it appears as a radiolucency superimposed with the apical portion of the maxillary central incisors. The anterior nasal spine visualized within the radiolucency may give it a heart-shape.

Various lesions to be considered in the differential diagnosis are large incisive foramen, radicular cyst, median palatine cyst, dentigerous cyst from a mesiodens or a primordial cyst from a supernumerary tooth.

Nasoalveolar Cyst

Nasoalveolar cyst is also called as the nasolabial cyst. It involves the soft tissues and the bone involvement is only secondary. It is considered to be a fissural cyst.

Median Palatine Cyst

Median palatine cyst is essentially similar to the nasopalatine cyst. It develops superiorly in the nasopalatine canal. It is very rare in occurrence, developing in the midline of the hard palate behind the premaxillae. It can produce expansion of the roof of the mouth.

Radiographically it is radiolucent, occurring behind the incisive canal in the premolar-molar area. The borders are hyperostotic.

Lesions to be considered in the differential diagnosis are the nasopalatine cyst and the radicular cyst.

Traumatic Bone Cyst

Traumatic bone cyst is also called as simple bone cyst, progressive bony cyst, blood cyst, solitary bone cyst, hemorrhagic bone cyst of the mandible or extravasation cyst. This is not a true cyst as it does not have an epithelial lining. Trauma in a young person is considered to be the etiological factor which results in hematoma formation. The hematoma undergoes disintegration and results in the cyst formation. The cyst contains blood, serosanguinous fluid, blood clot or giant cells. Sometimes it may not contain any solid material. The cyst can either expand or regress.

The borders of the cyst are ill-defined. In the radiograph it appears as an area of radiolucency conforming to the shape of the marrow space and occurring above the mandibular canal. The cyst is usually present in the mandibular posterior region. The cyst can project into the interdental bone and the ramus. If it occurs in the anterior region it may be round or oval.

History of trauma sustained during childhood may be helpful in the diagnosis. Aspiration may not provide anything or sometimes serosanguinous fluid or blood may be obtained.

The other lesions to be considered in the differential diagnosis are periapical cyst, periapical cementoma and median mandibular cyst.

Various treatment modalities that have been tried out in the management of this cyst are surgical opening to remove tissue debris and curettage of the bony wall to induce bleeding. Then the opening is closed. Another method involves injection of venous blood into the cavity.

Aneurysmal Bone Cyst

Aneurysmal bone cyst is not a true cyst as it does not have an epithelial lining. This cyst may be related to the traumatic bone cyst or the central giant cell granuloma. It is slow-growing and affects the mandible more predominantly than the maxilla. It mainly affects individuals less than 20 years of age. The cyst is slowly expansile. There can be missing or displaced teeth. Radiographically it appears either as a unilocular or multilocular lesion. Surgical curettage is the treatment of choice.

Odontogenic Tumors

I'm looking forward to a rough, rebellous, unrespectable old age,
Kicking the world uphill
With laughter shrill
And squeals of high-pitched, throaty rage.

– Don Marquis

INTRODUCTION

The odontogenic tumors originate due to the abnormal proliferation of cells and tissues of odontogenic origin. Some of the odontogenic tumors are characterized by their limited growth potential, whereas some represent true neoplasms.

A classification of the odontogenic tumors proposed by JJ Pindborg is given below.

Epithelial Odontogenic Tumors

A. Without inductive changes in connective tissue
 i. Ameloblastoma
 ii. Calcifying epithelial odontogenic tumor
B. With inductive changes in connective tissue
 i. Adenomatoid odontogenic tumor
 ii. Ameloblastic fibroma
 iii. Dentinoma
 iv. Odontoameloblastoma
 v. Odontomas
 – Ameloblastic fibro-odontoma
 – Complex odontoma
 – Compound odontoma.

Mesodermal Odontogenic Tumors

 i. Odontogenic fibroma
 ii. Odontogenic myxoma
 iii. Cementoma
 Periapical cemental dysplasia
 – Cementifying fibroma
 – Benign cementoblastoma
 – Gigantiform cementoma.

EPITHELIAL ODONTOGENIC TUMORS WITHOUT INDUCTIVE CHANGES

Ameloblastoma

The ameloblastoma is a true neoplasm without producing enamel. It contains ameloblasts differentiated from the ectodermal epithelium.

The tumor can arise from epithelial cells present in enamel organ, follicles, periodontal membrane, dentigerous cysts (mural ameloblastoma) and marrow spaces. Age of occurrence is in the third or fourth decade. There is no sex predilection. The common site of occurrence is the mandibular molar ramus area.

The classical radiographic appearance is multilocular cyst-like lesion of the jaw (Fig. 20-1). The multilocular appearance may be either of the honeycomb type or soap-bubble type. The lesion can cause resorption of roots of the teeth. If it occurs in the maxilla it produces a monocystic lesion. Sometimes even in the mandible the lesion can occur as a unilocular lesion.

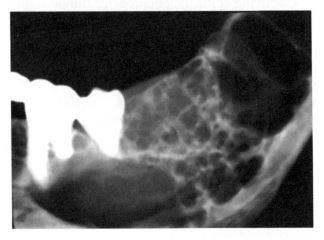

Fig. 20-1: Ameloblastoma of mandible

The tumor may be asymptomatic initially, later on becoming expansile and during this process the compartments may fuse together to form a large unilocular space. The tumor can also perforate the cortical plate.

The five histological types of ameloblastoma are:
- Simple or alveolar
- Plexiform
- Acanthomatous
- Spindle cell
- Granular cell.

The other lesions to be considered in the differential diagnosis are:

- Odontogenic keratocyst
- Dentigerous cyst
- Cementifying or ossifying fibroma
- Developmental bone defect
- Giant cell granuloma.

Surgical excision is the treatment of choice.

Calcifying Epithelial Odontogenic Tumor

Calcifying epithelial odontogenic tumor is also called as Pindborg's tumor. Some other names suggested for this tumor are calcifying ameloblastoma, malignant odontoma, and unusual ameloblastoma.

This tumor can occur at any age, but the common age of occurrence is about 40 years. The sex predilection is equal. The tumor occurs in the premolar or molar region. More lesions are reported in the maxilla than the mandible. Though the lesion is expansile, it does not expand into the interdental bone. A self-limiting feature of this tumor has been suggested due to the calcifications and amyloid-like substances found in the calcifying odontogenic tumor.

Treatment of this lesion is by surgery, but recurrence can occur.

EPITHELIAL ODONTOGENIC TUMORS WITH INDUCTIVE CHANGES (MIXED ODONTOGENIC TUMORS)

The mixed tumors are formed due to the proliferation of cells of ectodermal and mesodermal origin.

Adenomatoid Odontogenic Tumor (Adenoameloblastoma) (Fig. 20-2)

Adenomatoid odontogenic tumor accounts for 3% of all odontogenic tumors. This tumor is usually associated with unerupted teeth (Fig. 20-2). It can also occur independently. The age of occurrence is usually in the second decade of life.

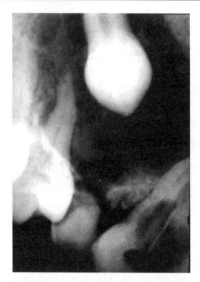

Fig. 20-2: Adenomatoid odontogenic tumor

Often it is detected during routine radiographic examination or in the radiographic evaluation of noneruption of the teeth. Varying degrees of calcification is seen within the tumor. These are rounded or structureless globules similar to cementicles. Though the lesion is expansile, local invasion is not seen.

Radiographically it appears as a unilocular lesion in association with an unerupted tooth. Areas of multiple radiopacities may be noted. Displacement of adjacent roots is a common finding. Radiographic appearance of this lesion is somewhat similar to that of odontogenic cysts. The lesions to be considered in the differential diagnosis are dentigerous cyst, keratinizing and calcifying odontogenic cyst, odontomas in the intermediate stage and calcifying epithelial odontogenic tumor.

The treatment of adenomatoid odontogenic tumor is by surgical enucleation and recurrence is very rare.

Ameloblastic Fibroma

Ameloblastic fibroma is a rare tumor developing from the dental follicle, after the onset of calcification of the tooth (Fig. 20-3). It can also develop in association with a tooth before the onset of calcification, resulting in the arrest of further tooth development. The epithelial cells mimic the primitive odontogenic epithelium. The typical histologic appearance is nests and cords of the odontogenic epithelium occurring in a myxomatous stroma.

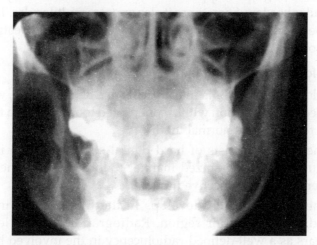

Fig. 20-3: Ameloblastic fibroma

Ameloblastic fibroma usually occurs in the posterior part of the jaws and the mandible is the most favored site. First two decades of life is the age of occurrence. The lesion has a benign clinical course and is slowly expansile. Radiographic appearance is uniform radiolucency with smooth well-defined borders. There may be septa within the lesion, causing a multilocular appearance. There can be displacement of roots of the teeth. Dentigerous cyst should be considered in the differential diagnosis. Treatment is by simple curettage.

Ameloblastic Sarcoma

Ameloblastic sarcoma is a rare odontogenic tumor. This tumor has also been called as malignant ameloblastoma, ameloblastosarcoma and ameloblastic fibrosarcoma. It is considered as a malignant counterpart of an ameloblastic fibroma.

Ameloblastic sarcoma predominantly occurs in the mandible. It is associated with rapid growth and pain. Swelling and paresthesia of the lips are some of the other features noted. It can occur at any age, between 15 to 75 years.

The radiographic appearance is a round radiolucency with irregular borders. Sometimes it also appears multilocular. There can be destruction of the bone. Surgical excision is the treatment of choice.

Ameloblastic Odontoma

Ameloblastic odontoma may arise from a dental follicle, when it is seen in association with an unerupted tooth or from a tooth bud, replacing the normal tooth.

The tumor consists of hard dental structures seen in an irregular and unorganized manner (odontogenic epithelium and embryonic connective tissue).

The tumor usually develops in the first decade, in the mandibular posterior region. Radiographically the lesion appears as a well-defined radiolucency in the involved bone, with even borders. Within the cavity varying amounts of radiopaque material is seen. There can also be a radiolucent component due to the presence of soft tissues.

The treatment of this lesion is by surgical enucleation.

Complex Odontoma

Complex odontoma originates similar to ameloblastic odontoma. The tumor consists of dentin, dentinoid, enamel, enamel matrix, pulp tissues and cementum in varying amounts and in an irregular pattern. The lesion is surrounded by a connective tissue capsule. The frequent site of occurrence is the mandibular premolar-molar region.

Radiographic examination reveals uniformly radiopaque mass in the proximity of the crown of an unerupted tooth. There is a radiolucent rim surrounding the lesion. The complex odontoma can also arise in relation to a supernumerary tooth. Treatment of complex odontoma is by surgical enucleation.

Compound Odontoma

The compound odontoma originates from the odontogenic epithelium, capable of producing enamel, resulting in the formation of small tooth-like structures. There can be varying number of tooth-like structures which undergo maturation. The common site of occurrence is the canine region. This lesion has also been reported in the premolar and third molar region as well as in the maxillary anterior region.

Radiographically, the lesion appears as an irregular mass within which tooth-like structures can be identified. On many situations, the compound odontoma is identified only during routine radiographic examination.

Dentinoma

Dentinoma is a rare odontogenic tumor, composed of dentin, soft tissue and cementum. The cementum is laid down in the periphery of the lesion. Very often this tumor is associated with the crown portion of unerupted permanent posterior teeth. Rarely the lesion can occur in association with the deciduous teeth.

The radiographic finding is that of a radiopaque mass in the region of the crown of an unerupted tooth.

MESODERMAL ODONTOGENIC TUMORS

Odontogenic Fibroma

Odontogenic fibroma may originate from the dental follicles, dental papilla or periodontal ligament. This is a rare odontogenic tumor. It occurs in the mandible of children and young adults. Treatment of odontogenic fibroma is by simple surgical means.

Odontogenic Myxoma

Odontogenic myxoma is also called as fibromyxoma. The jaw lesions are very rare. The lesion may originate from the undifferentiated embryonic tissue or from the mesenchymal portion of a tooth germ.

Both the jaws have equal preponderance. In the mandible, the molar region, the angle and the ramus are the frequent sites. In the maxilla, the zygomatic process and the premolar-molar regions are the favored sites. Clinically this tumor is noted as hard painless swellings. In some patients there can be facial asymmetry.

In the radiograph, the lesion appears as a well-defined radiolucency with multilocular compartments. The lesions to be considered in the differential diagnosis are ameloblastoma, giant cell granuloma and fibrous dysplasia.

This tumor is clinically benign, but locally invasive. The treatment involves enucleation and curettage or radical excision.

Cementifying Fibroma (Cementoma)

Cementifying fibroma is composed of mesenchymal elements. It is derived from the periodontal membrane of fully developed and erupted teeth.

Cementifying fibroma occurs more predominantly in the mandible than in the maxilla, as a result of connective tissue proliferation of the periodontal ligament. Initially a mass of fibrous tissue is produced and then there is formation of calcified bodies. There are three possible clinical course for this lesion.

a. The lesion remains as a peripheral fibroma or cemento-blastoma
b. The fibrous mass gets calcified and resembles cementum and normal bone
c. The fibrous tissue is replaced by bone.

The radiographic appearance is dependent on the stage of development of the lesion. In the early stage it appears as a uniform area of radiolucency. In the second stage there is calcified substance appearing within the radiolucency. In the third stage there is complete calcification of the lesion. There is a radiolucent space separating the calcified mass from the adjacent bone. This feature helps in differentiating it from idiopathic osteosclerosis, condensing osteitis and enostosis. Usually no surgical treatment is required as this lesion does not attain considerable size.

Gigantiform Cementoma

The gigantiform cementoma is a rare odontogenic tumor. It consists of benign lobulated mass of calcified, dense and acellular cementum. This lesion originates from the periodontal ligament. This tumor has also been termed as monstrous cementoma or florid osseous dysplasia. Radiographically it may not be possible to differentiate it from Paget's disease, chronic sclerosing osteomyelitis, osteopetrosis and multiple enostosis. It contains dense opaque material as seen in the radiograph.

Histologically these lesions contain cementum-like material. The lesions can have considerable growth in the second and third decade, resulting in cortical plate expansion.

Surgical treatment is carried out only for cosmetic purpose.

Chapter 21

Benign and Malignant Nonodontogenic Tumors of the Jaws

- *Introduction*
- *Benign Tumors*
  - *Exostosis and tori*
  - *Enostosis*
  - *Osteomas*
  - *Chondroma*
  - *Neurogenic tumors (neurilemoma, neurofibroma)*
  - *Peripheral fibroma with calcification*
  - *Central giant cell granuloma*
  - *Central hemangioma of bone*
- *Malignant Tumors*
  - *Carcinoma*
  - *Mucoepidermoid carcinoma*
  - *Sarcoma*
  - *Osteosarcoma or osteogenic sarcoma*
  - *Malignant lymphoma*
  - *Chondrosarcoma*
  - *Multiple myeloma*

And I know that this passes:
This implacable fury and torment of men,
As a thing insensate and vane:
And the stillness hath said unto me,
Over th tumult of sounds and shaken flame,
Out of the terrible beauty of wrath,
I alone am eternal.
One bough of clear promise
Across the moon.

– Frederic Manning

INTRODUCTION

As the name implies, nonodontogenic tumors do not originate from the odontogenic tissue. Many of the benign non-odontogenic tumors are harmless and are often detected on routine clinical examination, whereas, some of the malignant nonodontogenic tumors have an aggressive growth leading to destruction and disfigurement.

BENIGN TUMORS

Exostosis and Tori

Exostosis is a bony overgrowth or protuberance, usually seen on the facial surface of the jaws. Usually it has a smooth and uniform surface. The tori are essentially similar to the exostoses except that their locations are different. The term tori is used when the bony overgrowth is seen either in the midline of the palate or on the lingual surface of the mandible.

Torus palatinus is the bony protuberance occurring at the midline of the palate, involving both the sides of the borders of the suture line. Sometimes there may be a furrow or median groove over the bony protuberance. In some cases the lesion appears lobulated. The size of the lesion can vary considerably. A maxillary occlusal projection may be used for visualizing the torus palatinus. It is visualized as a localized area of radiopacity with well-defined borders (cortex). The inner portion of the torus may contain trabeculae. Though no treatment is required for torus palatinus, placement of maxillary denture may be difficult if the lesion is considerably larger.

Torus mandibularis is a bony protuberance occurring on the lingual surface of the mandible, especially in the premolar region. Often the mandibular tori are present bilaterally and above the mylohyoid ridge. The size varies. On radiographic examination, the mandibular tori can be visualized as a localized area of radiopacity. The symmetrical location and uniform outline help in the diagnosis.

No treatment is required for torus mandibularis unless it interferes with the placement of denture.

Enostosis

Unlike the exostosis, the enostosis originates from the inner surface of the cortical plate extending into the medullary space. Enostosis may not attain considerably larger size and is often detected on routine radiographic examination as localized area of radiopacity.

Osteomas

The osteomas are benign tumors originating from the bone. The size of the lesion may greatly vary from small to large. The larger lesions can cause cosmetic disfigurement. Some lesions exhibit a stalk (pedunculated), whereas other lesions are broad-based. The osteomas are more commonly seen involving the skull.

Osteoid osteoma is defined as a small, oval or roundish tumor-like nidus which is composed of osteoid and trabeculae of newly formed bone deposited within a substratum of highly vascularized osteogenic connective tissue. It usually occurs near the cortex and is very painful, usually seen in patients less than 30 years of age. The radiographic appearance is a radiopaque nidus surrounded by an irregular radiolucency which in turn is covered by bone of increased radiodensity.

The benign osteoblastoma is also called as giant osteoid osteoma. It can become quite large, but is less painful.

The osteomas can occur as a part of Gardner's syndrome.

Chondroma

The chondroma is a tumor of the cartilage. If it is partially ossified it is called osteochondroma, whereas if it is completely ossified it is called osteoma. It is a rare lesion affecting the jaws (it commonly occurs in the toes, fingers, sternum or the ribs). Radiographically it appears as a relatively radiolucent mass with areas of calcification. The bone is often sclerotic. There is a tendency for chondromas to undergo malignant transformation.

Neurogenic Tumors (Neurilemoma, Neurofibroma)

The neurogenic tumors can occur rarely in the jaws. The neurilemoma is encapsulated, whereas the neurofibroma is not. The neoplasm can occur in association with von Recklinghausen's disease or neurofibromatosis as cutaneous or subcutaneous tumors. The neurogenic tumors can occur at any age and there is no sex predilection. They are slow-growing lesions often causing neurologic symptoms such as paresthesia.

Radiographically they appear as radiolucency in association with the inferior alveolar canal. These lesions can also appear as multilocular cystic radiolucency resulting in extensive bone change, expansion or perforation of the cortical plates. A neurofibroma occurring near the surface of the bone can cause erosive areas of the bone.

Peripheral Fibroma with Calcification

The peripheral fibroma can originate from the periodontium, arising from the gingival crevice on the buccal, labial or lingual surface, usually less than 2 cm in diameter. The lesion usually has a large pedicle. Radiographically it appears as a radiopaque mass separate from the alveolar process. The degree of radiopacity differs based on the amount of calcification. Treatment of the lesion is by surgical excision.

Central Giant Cell Granuloma

The central giant cell granuloma is also called as benign giant cell tumor. The terminology of this lesion is highly debated. The current concept is to term this as giant cell lesion. The giant cell granuloma can occur either as a peripheral lesion or as a central lesion. The peripheral lesion can occur either in the maxilla or the mandible on the gingiva or the alveolar process, and is often pedunculated. Radiographically there may be involvement of the bone. If there is involvement of the bone, it may not be a deeper invasion.

The central giant cell granuloma usually occurs in children and young adults, below the age of 20 years. Females have a significantly greater predilection and the mandible is the most favored site. In the mandible, the usual site is anterior to the molars. The presence of swelling is variable and the lesion can cross the midline.

Radiographic picture may be either of a homogenous, osteolytic, monolocular lesion without any trabeculae with destructive areas of the cortex or multiple osteolytic areas and trabeculae with thinning and expansion of the cortex.

The treatment of central giant cell granuloma is by surgical curettage. Rarely recurrence is noted.

The jaw lesions of hyperparathyroidism are quite similar to the giant cell lesions. But it should be remembered that all the patients with hyperparathyroidism will not exhibit osseous changes in the jaws and all giant cell lesions are not associated with hyperparathyroidism.

Central Hemangioma of Bone

The hemangioma is a hamartoma. A hamartoma is defined as tumor-like malformation characterized by the presence of particular histologic tissue in improper proportions or distribution, with a prominent excess of one type of tissue. The hemangioma in the jaws are rare. The maxilla or the mandible may be involved in case of the jaw lesions. If it occurs in the jaws, bleeding from the gingival crevice and pumping action of the tooth (rebounding of the tooth when pushed into the socket) may be the clinical features. The other clinical features may be slowly progressing swelling of the jaw.

Radiographically the lesion appears to have cystic changes. The typical radiographic appearance is honeycomb pattern or it is multilocular with small multiple compartments of bone. In some cases the trabeculae appear to be extending from the center to the periphery.

As routine biopsy procedures can result in excessive bleeding, a needle aspiration should be carried out prior to biopsy in suspected cases.

MALIGNANT TUMORS

A malignant tumor in the jaws has a considerable growth potential at a faster rate leading to rapid destruction of the bone. The jaw lesions may be either primary or metastatic. Malignant jaw lesions usually have ill-defined borders. They grow by invasion and destruction of the neighboring structures. The jaw lesions are radiolucent unless there is new bone formation as seen in sarcoma.

Carcinoma

The squamous cell carcinoma is the commonest carcinoma affecting the oral cavity and involving the jaws. The invasion of the bone is a late finding. Initially there is erosion of the surface, proceeding to cause destruction of the cortex, and then widespread destruction of the bone. Radiographically, the lesion appears as an area of diffuse radiolucency. The borders are usually ill-defined. Rarely there can be expansion of the cortex. Severe destruction of the bone results in teeth with "hanging in space" appearance.

The metastatic jaw lesions usually involve the central area of the jaws as the red bone marrow is the most frequent site of metastasis. Initially there may be an osteolytic area which is not very specific for arriving at a diagnosis. There can be several associated complaints such as numbness of the lips and the chin region. In advanced cases there can be widespread destruction of the bone. The metastatic jaw lesions mainly originate from carcinoma of the breast. They can also originate from other sites. In some cases there can be bilateral involvement.

Mucoepidermoid Carcinoma

The mucoepidermoid carcinoma is a malignant lesion of the salivary glands. Rarely the tumor can occur as a central lesion either in the maxilla or the mandible in the premolar-molar area, usually in patients over 40 years of age. The radiographic appearance is cystic, often resembling dentigerous cyst. Complete surgical excision is the treatment.

Sarcoma

The sarcoma is a malignant tumor which originates from the connective tissues (fibrous tissue, cartilage, bone, muscle, fat or endothelial tissues). Most of the sarcomas are seen in young individuals. These lesions have metastatic tendency through the lymphatics. The radiographic examination plays a very useful role in the diagnosis of the jaw lesions, as diffuse areas of destruction. In some cases there can be excessive cartilage or bone deposition. Excessive bone deposition is visualized as areas of radiopacity.

The fibrosarcoma is a tumor of the spindle-shaped cells involving the jaws. Both the sexes and young and old individuals are affected in the same frequency. The radiographic appearance is localized alveolar bone destruction below a clinically observable swelling.

Osteosarcoma or Osteogenic Sarcoma

It is one of the frequently encountered primary tumor involving the jaw bones. It may arise from primitive undifferentiated cells and due to the malignant transformation of osteoblasts. An increased incidence of osteogenic sarcoma is seen in previously irradiated bone or bones with Paget's disease. This neoplasm usually occurs in individuals who are in their second or third decade of life, the range being second to fifth decades.

The clinical features may be pain, swelling, paresthesia mobility of the teeth, intraoral bleeding, facial asymmetry, or tissue mass in the alveolar ridge or in the gingiva. Some patients report with reddish, nodular growth from the socket of a recent extraction site. Males have a slightly greater predilection. The maxilla (alveolar ridge) or the mandible (body region) may be affected.

Radiographically, the lesion may be radiolucent, mixed radiolucent and radiopaque or predominantly radiopaque. The mixed lesion has ill-defined borders. These radiolucent-radiopaque areas represent excessive bone production and destruction. There can also be sequestration of bone appearing more radiopaque. When the periosteum is involved, there can be spicules of new bone directed outward producing the characteristic sunburst effect. Another radiographic appearance is 'cumulus cloud' formation. In some cases, two triangular radiopacities may project from the cortex (Codman's triangles). In some cases there may be periosteal deposition of bone, called onionskin appearance or band-like thickening of the lamina dura.

The lesions to be considered in the differential diagnosis are peripheral fibroma with calcification, ossifying subperiosteal hematoma, osteoblastic type of metastatic tumor or chondrosarcoma.

The treatment measures are radical and local surgery with radiotherapy, chemotherapy or combination therapy.

Malignant Lymphoma

The malignant lymphomas, also termed as reticulum cell sarcomas, originate from the lymphocytes and reticulum cells. The jaw lesions are rare, often involving the maxillae. The clinical features are swelling, pain and paresthesia. Radiographic examination reveals destructive areas. The treatment of lymphomas is either by radiotherapy or by chemotherapeutic drugs.

Chondrosarcoma

Chondrosarcoma of the jaws is a rare entity. It differs from osteosarcoma in clinical, therapeutic, and prognostic aspects. If these lesions involve the jaws, swelling, pain and paresthesia are the common complaints. The radiographic appearance may be suggestive of malignancy, but with varying degrees of calcification. The treatment of this lesion is by surgical excision.

Multiple Myeloma

Multiple myeloma is a plasma cell neoplasm. A solitary component or solitary myeloma is also existent. This neoplasm shows involvement of multiple skeletal sites such as the ribs, the sternum, the skull, the clavicles or the vertebral column. In the early stages small radiolucent areas in the bone marrow are seen. As these areas increase in number they may coalesce to form large irregular areas. The characteristic radiographic appearance is multiple punched-out osteolytic areas. There can also be involvement of the cortex.

Most of the jaw lesions involve the mandible. In some cases there is involvement of both the mandible and the maxilla. Usually the jaw lesions are bilateral.

The diagnosis is made by hyperglobulinemia, reversal of albumin-globulin ratio, increase in serum proteins and presence of Bence Jones proteins in the urine.

Fibro-Osseous Lesions

- *Introduction*
- *Fibrous Dysplasia*
- *Ossifying Fibroma*
- *Periapical Cemental Dysplasia*
- *Localized Fibro-osseous-cemental Lesions*
- *Florid Cemento-osseous Dysplasia*
- *Cementoblastoma*
- *Juvenile Aggressive Ossifying/Cementifying Fibroma*
- *Cherubism*
- *Paget's Disease (Osteitis Deformans)*

But they take not their courage from anger
That blinds the hot being;
They take not their pity from weakness;
Tender, yet seeing

– Laurence Binyon

INTRODUCTION

The fibro-osseous lesions are a diverse group of conditions that pose considerable difficulties in proper classification, categorization, and treatment. A common feature of all these lesions is that, there is replacement of the normal bone by a tissue composed of collagen fibers and fibroblasts that contain varying amounts of mineralized substances. The mineralized substances may be either osseous in nature, cementum-like, or combinations of bone or cementum.

The radiographic appearance of these lesions is also variable. These lesions may appear either as diffuse ground glass pattern or well-defined cystic areas that may be radiolucent or containing varying amounts of calcified material.

Fibro-osseous lesions have variously been classified and there is no consensus among the scientific community as to the categorization of various lesions belonging to this group.

A simple way of classifying the fibro-osseous lesions is to broadly divide these lesions into two groups based on their site of origin. Accordingly, the fibro-osseous lesions of periodontal ligament origin are cementifying fibroma, ossifying fibroma, cemento-ossifying fibroma and fibroma. The second group of fibro-osseous lesions originates from the medullary bone. These lesions are fibro-osteoma, active juvenile ossifying fibroma, fibrous dysplasia, giant cell tumor, aneurysmal bone cyst, jaw lesions associated with hyperparathyroidism, cherubism and Paget's disease.

A simple working classification of the fibro-osseous lesions is given below:

I. Fibrous dysplasia

II. Fibro-osseous (cemental) lesions of suspected periodontal ligament origin
   A. Periapical cemental dysplasia
   B. Localized fibro-osseous cemental lesion
   C. Florid cemento-osseous dysplasia (gigantiform cementoma)
   D. Ossifying and cementifying fibroma.

III. Fibro-osseous neoplasms of uncertain origin or those arising from the periodontal ligament
   A. Cementoblastoma, osteoblastoma, and osteoid osteoma
   B. Juvenile aggressive ossifying fibroma.

An important aspect to be noted in this classification is that the concept of medullary bone origin is not accepted. In short, it should be stressed that, there is no acceptable classification for these so-called fibro-osseous lesions.

As most of the lesions belonging to this diverse group are discussed elsewhere, only selected lesions will be discussed in this chapter.

FIBROUS DYSPLASIA

The term fibrous dysplasia was proposed by Lichtenstein in 1938. Fibrous dysplasia is a benign fibro-osseous lesion (Fig. 22-1). Its origin is not properly known. It is assumed that this lesion originates from the medullary bone. Two types of fibrous dysplasia have been recognized, the monostotic or the solitary form and the polyostotic form. The polyostotic form involves multiple bones and is usually unilateral.

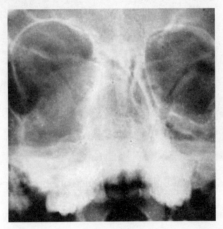

Fig. 22-1: Fibrous dysplasia involving the maxillary sinus

Albright's syndrome is characterized by pigmentation of the skin, precocious puberty and polyostotic fibrous dysplasia in females.

Fibrous dysplasia predominantly involves the maxilla than the mandible and is unilateral. The tumor usually manifests between 10–30 years of age. Often the posterior region of the jaw is involved. The presenting complaints are hard swelling, facial asymmetry and malocclusion. The swelling is slow-growing over a period of time.

The radiographic appearance can vary depending on the stage of the lesion. In lesions with more fibrous tissue, it may appear as radiolucency, either unilocular or multilocular. Lesions with osseous tissue have a mottled appearance. Lesions with excessive osseous tissue appear radiopaque. The typical radiographic appearance is termed as 'ground glass' or 'orange peel' appearance (Fig. 22-2). Usually the lesion is well-circumscribed.

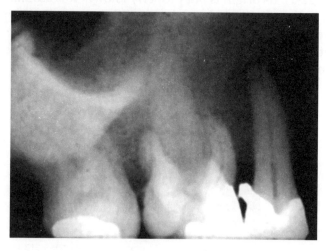

Fig. 22-2: Ground glass appearance of fibrous dysplasia

The treatment of fibrous dysplasia is by surgery for cosmetic purpose.

OSSIFYING FIBROMA

Ossifying fibroma, a rare neoplasm, is also called as fibro-osteoma. It is an encapsulated lesion within which the highly cellular fibrous tissue undergoes calcification. Though ossifying fibroma is locally aggressive, it is not considered malignant. It usually affects young adults. Females have a slightly greater predilection. The lesion is slow-growing and causes displacement of the teeth. Usually it involves the mandible and presents in the premolar-molar region. In the maxilla it is found in the canine fossa and the zygomatic process regions.

Radiographic findings depend on the stage of development of the lesion. It may either appear radiolucent or multiple radiopaque foci may be seen within the radiolucency. Eventually these foci coalesce together. Borders of the lesion are well-defined, often showing radiolucent rim suggestive of fibrous capsule. There may be displacement of the teeth.

Other lesions to be considered in the differential diagnosis are adenomatoid odontogenic tumor, osteogenic sarcoma, and fibrous dysplasia.

Table 22-1 shows the differences between fibrous dysplasia and ossifying fibroma.

Table 22-1: Differences between fibrous dysplasia and ossifying fibroma

Fibrous dysplasia	Ossifying fibroma
Borders are ill-defined	Borders are well-defined
Root resorption not usually seen	Root resorption is common
Homogeneous radiopaque area	Radiolucent or radiopaque
Granular appearance	Radiolucent with radiopaque specks
Treated by bone shaving for cosmetic purposes	Completely removed

PERIAPICAL CEMENTAL DYSPLASIA

Periapical cemental dysplasia was earlier called as cementoma. It is also variously named as fibrocementoma, sclerosing cementoma, periapical osteofibrosis, or periapical fibro-osteosis. It is considered as a reactive fibro-osseous lesion.

The lesion usually occurs in the middle age and females are affected more than the males. There is a tendency for the lesion to occur in the blacks. The lesion usually occurs in the periapical region of the mandibular anterior teeth and the lesions may be multiple. The affected teeth are vital. Periapical cemental dysplasia is an asymptomatic lesion and most often is detected during a routine radiographic examination.

Radiographic appearance of the lesion depends on the stage of development of the lesion. Accordingly, it may be radiolucent (fibrous), mixed radiolucent-radiopaque (fibrous and calcified elements), or radiopaque (calcified stage). The margins of the lesion may be well-defined or ill-defined.

Lesions to be considered in the differential diagnosis are periapical condensing osteitis, complex odontoma and benign cementoblastoma. Usually no treatment is required for periapical cemental dysplasia.

LOCALIZED FIBRO-OSSEOUS-CEMENTAL LESIONS

This group of fibro-osseous lesions are ill-defined and are difficult to classify. The clinical and radiographic findings of these lesions are quite different from that of periapical cemental dysplasia and florid cemento-osseous dysplasia. As these lesions do not possess growth potential, they are not considered to be neoplastic. The lesion is usually solitary. The radiographic features depend on the stage of development of the lesion. Thus the radiographic appearance may be radiolucent, mottled pattern of mixed radiolucency and radiopacity or largely radiopaque. The lesion is usually spotted in the mandibular posterior region. Most often the lesion is asymptomatic and does not cause cortical plate expansion. As most of the lesions are located at the site of previous extraction or in edentulous patients, an abnormal reaction of the bone to trauma has been suggested.

Histologically, the lesion contains fibrous tissue and varying amounts of calcified material; either bone, cementum or combination of both bone and cementum.

FLORID CEMENTO-OSSEOUS DYSPLASIA

Florid osseous dysplasia is also called as gigantiform cementoma, chronic sclerosing osteomyelitis, sclerosing osteitis, multiple enostosis, and sclerotic cemental mass. Florid cemento-osseous dysplasia is similar to periapical cemental dysplasia.

This lesion has a female predilection, usually occurring in the middle-age. Both the jaws are usually involved simultaneously. Sometimes it occurs only in the mandible. Often the lesion does not cause any symptoms. Occasionally pain or swelling may be noted. A great majority of the patients are edentulous or partially edentulous during initial presentation. The tissue from the lesion consists of dense, sclerotic masses that are similar to cementum. Though some workers consider this tissue to be bone, several histochemical and electron microscopic studies have shown that the nature of this tissue is more similar to cementum.

Radiographically the lesion appears radiolucent with dense radiopaque masses within. It has a similarity to "cotton-wool" appearance of Paget's disease. Individual lesions often exhibit a cortical outline.

Some lesions to be considered in the differential diagnosis are Paget's disease and osteopetrosis.

CEMENTOBLASTOMA

Cementoblastoma is a rare neoplasm originating in the periodontal ligament. Males have a greater predilection and usually occurs before 25 years of age. Mandible is the favored site and it appears as a solitary lesion. The involved tooth is vital. The tumor is slow-growing and forms a mass at the root. Rarely expansion of the jaws can occur.

Radiographically it appears as a well-defined radiopacity at the apex of a premolar or molar. Usually the calcified mass shows radiolucent halo.

Various other lesions to be considered in the differential diagnosis are periapical cemental dysplasia, chronic focal sclerosing osteomyelitis, periapical osteosclerosis and hypercementosis.

JUVENILE AGGRESSIVE OSSIFYING/CEMENTIFYING FIBROMA

Though some lesions have been reported in the literature as juvenile aggressive ossifying/cementifying fibroma, there is no clear demarcation between this lesion and the more common ossifying/cementifying fibroma.

Most of the cases of aggressive juvenile ossifying fibroma have been reported in the maxilla, in patients who are in the first or second decades of life. This lesion exhibits a cellular nature and produces only scanty collagen. There is formation of osteoid and there is abundant numbers of giant cells.

CHERUBISM

Cherubism is characterized by bilateral benign, firm, painless swellings in the mandible, usually in the angle region. Other sites are also involved. If it occurs in the maxilla, it is usually seen in the tuberosity region. The lesion usually develops in the infancy and continues to grow causing greatest expansion in the first and second years after the onset. As the age advances the deformity becomes less obvious. The lesion has a familial tendency.

The lesion has derived the name as the affected children have characteristic chubby, cherubic facial appearance. Typically, the affected individuals have "eyes raised to the heaven" appearance, if the lesion involves the maxilla.

The characteristic radiographic appearance is multiple cyst-like radiolucencies in the mandible. The lesions have multilocular appearance and the borders are well-defined. Cortical plate expansion is seen in the occlusal or PA views. Maxillary lesions project into the maxillary sinus. The developing tooth buds are usually displaced. There is usually premature exfoliation of the deciduous teeth.

Various lesions to be considered in the differential diagnosis are fibrous dysplasia, giant cell granuloma and aneurysmal bone cyst.

As the lesion is self-limiting, no treatment is required.

PAGET'S DISEASE (OSTEITIS DEFORMANS)

Paget's disease was described as a clinical entity by Sir James Paget in 1877 and is characterized by abnormal bone destruction followed by bone formation involving several bones. One concept regarding the origin of this disease is that it is a slow virus infection.

Though this disease mainly affects the skull, the femur, the sacrum and the pelvis, jaw involvement is rarely seen bilaterally. The incidence of the disease usually occurs above 50 years of age. Males are affected more than the females. Symptoms of the lesion are bone pain, increased temperature, curvature of the spine, enlargement of the skull and facial bones and bone deformity. In dentulous patients there can be drifting of the teeth and malocclusion. Edentulous patients often complain of ill-fitting dentures.

Serum alkaline phosphatase level is increased in these patients.

Radiographic appearance of this lesion depends on the stage of formation. Accordingly, it may be radiolucency of granular or 'ground glass' appearance or dense radiopaque or the so-called 'cotton wool' appearance. In the skull, the early lesions are lytic and appear as multiple radiolucencies called osteoporosis circumscripta.

Various lesions to be considered in the differential diagnosis are:
• Fibrous dysplasia
• Osteopetrosis
• Osteosclerosis
• Tori
• Osteomas.

The management of this lesion is done with calcitonin or sodium etidronate therapy. Surgery is indicated for cosmetic purposes.

Radiographic Features of Systemic Diseases

Never, never may the fruit be gathered from the bough
And harvested in barrels.
The winter of love is a cellar of empty bins,
In an orchard soft with rot.

– Edna St. Vincent May

DISORDERS OF THE ENDOCRINE SYSTEM

There are a variety of endocrine disorders with manifestations in the teeth and the jaws. These changes in the mineralized structures are apparent on radiographic examination. The involvement of the teeth and the jaws also depend on the time of occurrence of the endocrine disturbance with reference to the development of the involved structures. Endocrine disturbances during the period of growth and maturation may be manifested as retarded or accelerated facial development.

Disorders of the Pituitary Gland

Apart from the growth hormone, the pituitary gland secretes several hormones that have influence on the other endocrine glands. In hypopituitarism, the growth of the skeletal and the somatic tissues are affected leading to stunted growth. The facial growth is retarded. There can be growth retardation in the posterior facial height than in the anterior facial height. There is retardation of the formation, the calcification and the eruption of the teeth. The carpal maturation is also affected.

In hyperpituitarism, there is increased growth of somatic and skeletal tissues. Hyperpituitarism can result from adenoma of the pituitary gland or due to idiopathic factors. Hyperpituitarism in childhood or adolescence results in gigantism. The radiographic findings may be hypercementosis, spacing between the teeth, increase in dental arch size, increase in radiographic density, enlarged cranium or prognathic mandible. Acromegaly results due to hyperpituitarism in an adult. The radiographic features are enlargement of the mandible, endochondral-like growth of the condyle can result in increase in the height of the ramus and anterior and inferior positioning of the mandibular body and the symphysis. The associated macroglossia can result in flaring of the anterior teeth and spacing. Intraoral periapical radiographs may reveal hypercementosis.

Disorders of the Thyroid Gland

The thyroid gland secretes two very essential hormones, thyroxine and calcitonin. Thyroxine helps in the normal growth and maturation, whereas, calcitonin is essential for calcium homeostasis as it has a hypocalcemic action. Hypothyroidism results in cretinism in children and myxedema in adults. The radiographic features of hypothyroidism are decrease in facial height, retardation in the facial growth pattern, decreased cranial base length and increased flexion of the cranial base. There can be retarded development and eruption of dentition.

Hyperthyroidism is characterized by accelerated osseous development. The radiographic features are increase in the anterior facial growth leading to open-bite, there may be mandibular prognathism and increase in cranial base length. In some cases accelerated formation, calcification and eruption of the teeth may occur.

Disorders of the Parathyroid Gland

Hyperparathyroidism

In hyperparathyroidism there is excessive levels of parathyroid hormone (PTH) in circulation, resulting in hypercalcemia due to mobilization of calcium from the skeleton. PTH also enhances renal tubular reabsorption of calcium. Hyperparathyroidism is of three types:

- Primary hyperparathyroidism
- Secondary hyperparathyroidism
- Tertiary hyperparathyroidism

Primary hyperparathyroidism occurs due to a benign tumor or hyperplasia of the parathyroid gland resulting in excessive production of PTH. Diagnosis is often made by hypercalcemia and excessive circulating levels of PTH.

Secondary hyperparathyroidism occurs secondary to other factors that are responsible for hypocalcemia such as renal diseases, dietary deficiency or improper absorption. Hypocalcemia results in excessive production of PTH.

Tertiary hyperparathyroidism occurs due to hyperplasia of the parathyroid gland secondary to renal diseases.

Hyperparathyroidism affects the females more than the males (male to female ratio is 1:3). The average age of occurrence is between 30 and 60 years. The signs and symptoms of hyperparathyroidism are due to hypercalcemia such as bone and joint problems, renal stones, psychiatric problems and peptic ulcer. There may be jaw lesions as part of osteitis cystica generalisata. Loosening, drifting and loss of the teeth can occur.

Radiographic features of hyperparathyroidism are demineralization or pathologic calcifications. Only a few patients with hyperparathyroidism manifest bone changes. About 10% of cases manifest loss of the lamina dura in the periapical radiographs.

Hypoparathyroidism and Pseudohypoparathyroidism

In hypoparathyroidism there is low levels of circulating PTH. Hypoparathyroidism mainly results from accidental removal of the gland during surgical procedures involving the thyroid gland. In pseudohypoparathyroidism there is defective response by the target organs or tissues to normal levels of PTH. The clinical features are the result of hypocalcemia such as carpopedal spasm due to tetany, paresthesia of the hands and the feet, anxiety, depression or chorea. In chronic forms there can be calcification in the brain. The chief radiographic finding is calcification of the ganglia. Some of the discernible dental changes may be enamel hypoplasia, root resorption or altered eruption pattern (eruption is delayed).

Diabetes Mellitus

Diabetes mellitus (DM) is a metabolic disorder due to the deficiency of insulin. Two types of DM occurring in affected patients are:

- Type I or insulin-dependent (juvenile) DM
- Type II or noninsulin-dependent (maturity onset) DM.

Insulin is produced by the beta cells of the islets of Langerhans in the pancreas. A fall in the level of insulin adversely affects carbohydrate metabolism, leading to hyperglycemia and glycosuria.

The cardinal symptoms and signs of DM are

- Polyphagia (excessive food intake)
- Polydipsia (excessive fluid intake)

- Polyuria (excessive urination)
- Acetone in breath and urine due to ketoacidosis
- Decreased resistance to infection
- Neurological problems.

As diabetic patients are more prone for periodontal disease, there can be bone loss as visualized in dental radiographs. Clinically these patients manifest periodontal disease and/ or multiple periodontal abscesses. Infection of the socket after extraction can result in focal sclerosing osteomyelitis or dry socket.

Disorders of the Adrenal Gland

Cushing's Syndrome

Cushing's syndrome is the result of excessive glucocorticoid secretion by the adrenal glands. Usually hyperfunctioning of the adrenal glands occurs due to a neoplastic process. The females are affected more than the males.

Various clinical features of Cushing's syndrome are trunkal obesity, kyphosis of the thoracic spine, weakness, hypertension or striae. The characteristic radiographic finding is generalized osteoporosis. There is inhibition of bone deposition, but bone resorption continues. There can also be pathologic fractures. There is usually thinning of the skull and loss of the lamina dura.

METABOLIC DISORDERS

Idiopathic Histiocytosis (Langerhans cell disease)

Idiopathic histiocytosis or Langerhans cell disease was formerly known as histiocytosis X. It is a disorder characterized by proliferation of cells exhibiting phenotypic characteristics of Langerhans cells. This results in solitary or multiple bone lesions or disseminated visceral, skin and bone lesions.

Idiopathic histiocytosis comprises of three entities:

   i Letterer-Siwe disease
   ii Hand-Schüller-Christian disease
   iii Eosinophilic granuloma.

Letterer-Siwe Disease

Letterer-Siwe disease is also called as the acute disseminated form of Langerhans cell disease. It occurs in children below 3 years of age. Soft tissue and bony granulomatous lesions are disseminated throughout the body. The clinical features are fever, enlargement of the liver and the spleen, anemia, lymphadenopathy, hemorrhages and inability to thrive. Bone lesions are relatively rare. The disease is fatal.

Hand-Schüller-Christian Disease

Hand-Schüller-Christian disease is also called as the chronic disseminated form of Langerhans cell disease. Though the disease is initiated early in the childhood, it becomes apparent only in the third decade. The typical triad of abnormalities are bone lesions, diabetes insipidus and exophthalmos. The clinical course of the disease is variable with periods of remission and exacerbation.

Eosinophilic Granuloma

The term eosinophilic granuloma is used only if solitary or multiple bone lesions are present. The bony sites involved are the ribs, pelvis, the flat bones of the skull and the face and the long bones. It can also involve the lymph nodes, the skin, and the lungs. Involvement of the oral cavity can affect the gingiva and the palate.

The radiographic changes in eosinophilic granuloma are mainly seen in the skull. The lesions may be solitary or multiple. Jaw lesions are predominantly seen in the mandible than the maxilla. Jaw lesions are characterized by osteolysis and ultimately leading to "teeth standing in space" or "floating teeth" appearance. The lesions have "punched-out" appearance. Jaw lesions can be visualized more accurately by ^{99m}Tc-labeled diphosphate bone scan.

Various jaw lesions to be considered in the differential diagnosis are squamous cell carcinoma, giant cell lesions of the jaws, primordial and traumatic cysts, periodontal disease and cherubism.

Osteoporosis

Osteoporosis is characterized by decrease in the density of the bone, but with normal histological characteristics. Primary osteoporosis occurs as a result of aging process and is more predominantly seen in females. Secondary osteoporosis occurs secondary to other factors such as malnutrition or scurvy and corticosteroid or heparin therapy.

The affected individuals are more prone for fracture. Pathologic fractures are seen in the weight-bearing bones such as the spine or the hip in postmenopausal women. Estrogen therapy after menopause can prevent cortical and trabecular bone loss.

Radiographic features are thinning of the cortical plates, reduction in the density and thickness of the cortical plates, loss of the lamina dura, reduction in the trabecular pattern and stepladder pattern of the interdental trabeculae.

Rickets and Osteomalacia

Rickets and osteomalacia result from deficiency of vitamin D. The extracellular levels of calcium and inorganic phosphate are inadequate. Rickets affects infants and children, whereas osteomalacia affects adults. Often the deficiency of vitamin D is due to inadequate exposure to the sunlight. Gastrointestinal malabsorption can result in defective absorption of dietary vitamin D. Chronic renal and liver diseases and anticonvulsant therapy can also interfere with vitamin D absorption. Hypophosphatemic rickets is the term given for renal loss of inorganic phosphate without any alteration in calcium metabolism.

In children with rickets, tetany and convulsions can occur due to hypocalcemia, especially in the initial 6 months of age. Later on there can be other bone changes such as softening of the parietal bones (craniotabes), bony enlargement of the wrists and the ankles, deformities and short stature. A dental change which may be noted is delayed eruption of the teeth.

Osteomalacia is often associated with pain. Other features are muscle weakness, waddling or "penguin" gait, tetany and greenstick fractures.

Radiographically, rickets is characterized by widening of the epiphyses of long bones and bowing of weight-bearing long bones. There can be thinning of the cortical plates and reduction in the number of trabeculae. Enamel formation may be affected leading to hypoplasia, especially if the disorder occurs before 3 years of age.

Though thinning of the bone may not be a typical feature of osteomalacia, there can be poorly calcified ribbon-like zone (pseudofracture) extending into the bone at right angles especially in the ribs, the pelvis and the weight-bearing bones. Radiographs may reveal generalized radiolucent areas, sparse and course trabeculae and thinning of the lamina dura. The structure of the teeth is not usually affected.

Hypophosphatasia

Hypophosphatasia is an inherited disorder and the affected patients have low levels of serum alkaline phosphatase activity and high urinary excretion of phosphoethanolamine. In hypophosphatasia there is defective bone matrix formation.

Inheritance of this disorder may be of two ways; homozygous and heterozygous. Homozygous patients usually die soon after the birth. Such patients have defective skull formation and bowed limbs. Death occurs due to chest infections. Heterozygous patients show retarded growth and tendency for fracture.

The typical radiographic features are irregular defects of the long bones and decreased calcification of the skull. There may be multiple radiolucent areas in the skull radiographs due to gyral markings. These markings are called "beaten copper" appearance. Generalized radiolucency can affect the maxilla and the mandible. Tooth formation is adversely affected, characterized by reduced thickness of the enamel and enlarged pulp chambers and root canals.

Hypophosphatemia

Hypophosphatemia is also called as vitamin D-resistant rickets and is a genetic disorder. There is excessive renal loss of phosphorus. As the disease is transmitted in an X-linked dominant manner, the female patients transmit the disease to one-half of their offspring regardless of their sex. Male patients in turn transmit the disease to all their daughters and none of their sons.

Affected individuals manifest growth retardation and bony defects such as bowing of the legs, enlarged epiphyses and skull changes.

Radiographic features are similar to rickets, characterized by deformity, fractures or pseudofractures.

Renal Osteodystrophy

In renal osteodystrophy, there is a defect in the hydroxylation of 25-hydroxycholecalciferol (25-HCC) to 1, 25-dihydroxy-cholecalciferol (1,25-DHCC)due to chronic renal failure. The affected individuals have hypocalcemia due to defective calcium absorption and hyperphosphatemia due to decreased renal phosphorus excretion. The hypocalcemia leads to secondary hyperparathyroidism.

The clinical features are growth retardation, fractures, and signs of chronic renal failure.

The radiographic features are generalized loss of density of the bone, thinning of the cortical bone, loss of the lamina dura and poor bone growth in children. There is increase in the medullary space and scanty trabeculation.

DISORDERS OF THE BLOOD AND HEMATOPOIETIC SYSTEM

Sickle Cell Anemia

Sickle cell anemia is an inherited disorder characterized by abnormal hemoglobin which results in a tendency for sickling of the red blood cells (RBCs), when the oxygen tension is low. The oxygen carrying capacity is also reduced. The abnormal

RBCs can block the capillaries because of their adhesion to the endothelium. In the spleen the RBCs are readily destroyed and anemia ensues. This causes compensatory hyperplasia of the bone marrow at the expense of the spongy bone. Homozygous and heterozygous forms of this disorder have been recognized.

The clinical features during a crisis are muscle and joint pains, increase in temperature, weakness and circulatory collapse. During milder periods there can be weakness and shortness of breath. The heart may be enlarged with murmur. Many affected individuals die before 40 years of age because of the several associated complications.

Radiographic changes are due to hyperplasia of the bone marrow. There is thinning of the trabeculae and widening of diploe of the skull with thinning of the inner and outer tables. Loss of the outer table can result in hair-on-end appearance. Hypovascularity can lead to osteomyelitis in the jaws. The jaws also may demonstrate bone loss.

Thalassemia

Thalassemia or Cooley's anemia is a hereditary disorder associated with defect in hemoglobin synthesis. It can affect either the alpha or the beta chain of hemoglobin. The affected red blood cells have a low hemoglobin content and are short-lived. The heterozygous form is called thalassemia minor and the homozygous form is called thalassemia major. In the severe form the disorder manifests at infancy with a fatal outcome. Affected individuals have prominent cheekbones and protruded premaxillae.

Radiographic features are due to expansion of the bone marrow as part of compensatory mechanism. There is generalized radiolucency and thinning of the cortical plates. The diploe of the skull is widened. The skull usually has a granular appearance with a radial striation (hair-on-end appearance). Jaw changes are radiolucent areas, thinning of the cortical plates and large and course trabeculae. The lamina dura may become thin and the root length may be reduced as seen in the periapical radiographs. The prominent premaxillae can cause malocclusion.

The radiographic features are quite typical of this disease and the diagnosis is made by the radiographic findings. The typical radiographic appearance is bilaterally symmetrical increase in the density of the bone. The trabecular pattern is not radiographically discernible. There is increase in diameter of the long bones and they appear funnel-shaped due to the lack of remodeling.

Some of the dental changes noted are missing teeth, delayed eruption, early loss of teeth and malformation of teeth.

Some of the lesions to be considered in the differential diagnosis are infantile-cortical hyperostosis and osteogenic sarcoma.

BONE DISEASE OF UNKNOWN ORIGIN

Osteogenesis Imperfecta (Fragilitas ossium)

The etiology of osteogenesis imperfecta is unknown and it affects the mesodermal tissues. Two types of this disease have been noted, congenita or Vrolik's type and tarda or Lobstein's type. The affected individuals will have fragile bones that are more prone for fracture. Some of the clinical features are blue sclera, deafness and laxity of the ligaments. Osteogenesis imperfecta is often associated with dentinogenesis imperfecta. Some of the radiographic features are thinning of the cortex and loss of density of the bone.

REACTIVE LESIONS

Central Giant Cell Granuloma

Central giant cell granuloma is a nonneoplastic disease of the bone. It occurs in individuals below 20 years of age. The frequent site of occurrence is the mandible, usually anterior to the first molars. The lesion usually does not cause any symptoms and is often noticed as an enlargement resulting in facial asymmetry.

Radiographically the lesion appears as multilocular radiolucency with undulated and well-defined borders. Within the lesion there are wispy trabeculae. Maxillary lesions can erode the walls of the maxillary sinus or cause expansion of the bone. There can be displacement of adjacent tooth roots and tooth follicles.

Various other lesions to be considered in the differential diagnosis are ameloblastoma, odontogenic myxoma, aneurysmal bone cyst and ossifying fibroma.

HEREDITARY DISEASES

There are a wide variety of jaw diseases that may have a hereditary origin.

Osteopetrosis (Albers-Schönberg disease or Marble bone disease)

Osteopetrosis is a hereditary disease characterized by general increase in the bone density due to defective bone remodeling mechanism. Many of the milder cases are asymptomatic. Severe form of this disease is associated with bone pain and fractures. The affected individuals have a high incidence of osteomyelitis. Some of the other complications are cranial neuropathies, hydrocephalus, epilepsy and mental retardation.

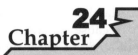

Chapter 24

Pathologic Soft Tissue Calcification

- *Introduction*
- *Lymph Nodes*
- *Sialolith*
- *Antrolith*
- *Calcified Stylohyoid Ligament*
- *Osteoma*
- *Calcified Blood Vessel*
- *Myositis Ossificans*
- *Cysticercosis*
- *Dystrophic Calcification*

A thousand rivers, lakes and seas
Hold up their mirrors to her gaze;
A thousand moonlets there she sees
Float on a thousand starry ways.

– Gerald Miller

INTRODUCTION

Soft tissue calcification refers to abnormal deposition of calcium and phosphate ions in an unorganized manner within the soft tissues.

A variety of pathologic processes can cause abnormal calcification of the soft tissues of the body that do not show any calcification under normal circumstances. Soft tissue calcification is associated with inflammatory conditions, infections, tumors or scars. The calcified material deposited is mainly calcium and phosphate ions.

LYMPH NODES

Among the soft tissues, calcification of lymph nodes is more prevalent. It is usually the result of chronic infections such as tuberculosis.

Radiographically a calcified lymph node appears radiopaque, sometimes with a laminated appearance. Either a single lymph node will be affected or multiple lymph nodes may be affected. The lymph nodes usually affected are the submandibular and the cervical lymph nodes.

A sialolith should be differentiated from a calcified lymph node. Often the associated clinical symptoms such as pain helps to differentiate a sialolith from a calcified lymph node. Usually the calcified lymph nodes do not require any treatment.

SIALOLITH

A sialolith is a calcareous matter occurring within the major or the minor salivary glands or their ducts. Sialoliths occur more predominantly in the submandibular salivary gland and its duct. Sialoliths are associated with pain especially before the mealtime.

Mandibular occlusal radiograph is very helpful in the identification of calculi within the submandibular gland or its duct. Radiographically, it appears as a small, round or oval radiopacity. Sialography is another investigative procedure in the diagnosis of a sialolith. Sialography demonstrates filling defect distal to the obstruction. There may be ductal dilatation proximal to the site of obstruction due to the collection of the contrast agent used for sialography. Removal of a sialolith either by manual manipulation or by surgical excision is necessary in the management. Only superficial sialoliths within the duct can be removed by manipulation.

ANTROLITH

Antroliths are calcified masses occurring within the maxillary antrum. Usually antroliths originate from the calcification of accumulated mucus, root fragments, bone fragments or foreign objects. The size and density of the calcified mass may vary. Antroliths should be differentiated from displaced root fragments into the maxillary sinus.

CALCIFIED STYLOHYOID LIGAMENT

Calcification of the stylohyoid ligament is commonly seen in panoramic radiographs, even in many asymptomatic patients. Eagles' syndrome is a term given for elongated stylohyoid ligament associated with pain.

Based on the pattern of calcification and the appearance of the styloid process, elongated and mineralized stylohyoid ligament is classified into different types. The classification based on the pattern of calcification is represented in Figure 24-1.

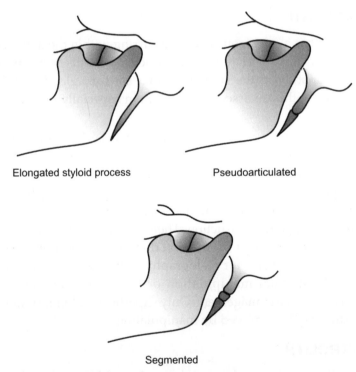

Elongated styloid process   Pseudoarticulated

Segmented

Fig. 24-1: Elongated styloid process

Classification of elongated styloid process based on the appearance is given below:

A. i. Slightly elongated
ii. Crooked
iii. Segmented
iv. Very elongated
B. Type I Elongated (normally, 25 to 32 mm)
Type II Pseudoarticulated
Type III Segmented
C. Based on the pattern of calcification (Fig. 24-2)
i. A calcified outline
ii. Partially calcified
iii. A nodular complex
iv. Completely calcified.

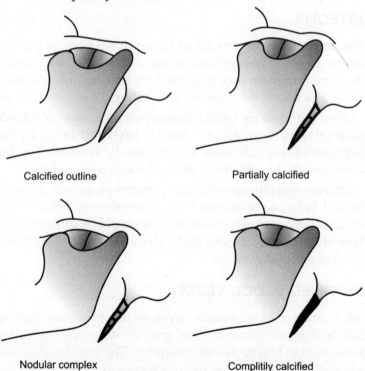

Calcified outline

Partially calcified

Nodular complex

Complitily calcified

Fig. 24-2: Classification of elongated stylohyoid ligament based on the pattern of calcification

The common symptoms associated with elongated stylohyoid ligament are pain on swallowing, turning the head, or opening the mouth. There can also be headache, dizziness, earache or occasional syncope. These symptoms are associated with compression of the styloid process on the glosso-pharyngeal nerve (V cranial nerve).

In the radiograph, styloid process appears as a long, thin, pointed radiopaque structure seen between the ramus of the mandible and the mastoid process. It usually tapers from the base. In a panoramic radiograph, the mineralized stylohyoid ligament should have 29 mm to be called as elongated styloid process.

In symptomatic patients, surgical removal can be carried out.

OSTEOMA

Osteoma cutis is the process of laying down bone in the soft tissues. Face is a common site of occurrence of osteoma cutis. The bone formation occurs in the dermis or the subcutaneous tissue. The size of the osteoma varies from 0.1 mm to 5.0 mm.

Often the cause for facial osteomas are acne, scars or chronic inflammatory dermatoses. Needle insertion helps in the diagnosis of this condition. When a needle is inserted in the suspected site of osteoma, a stone-like resistance is felt.

On radiographic examination, osteomas appear as well-defined radiopaque masses with a radiolucent center which contains fatty marrow. Osteoma cutis should be differentiated from myositis ossificans and calcinosis cutis. Treatment involves surgical excision.

CALCIFIED BLOOD VESSEL

Calcification of blood vessels can occur due to arteriosclerosis. Calcification can occur in facial arteries. Arterial calcification is also seen in Sturge-Weber syndrome. The associated cranial hemangiomas often show high incidence of calcification. The calcified vessel usually appears as thin radiopaque lines in the radiograph.

MYOSITIS OSSIFICANS

Myositis ossificans refers to replacement of muscle with ossifying tissue. Two types of myositis ossificans have been recognized, localized or traumatic myositis ossificans and progressive myositis ossificans.

Localized myositis ossificans is usually the result of traumatic injuries or heavy muscular strain. The possible chain of events can be summarized as given below.

Chain of events in the origin of myositis ossificans (Flow chart 24-1)

Flow chart 24-1: Development of myositis ossificans

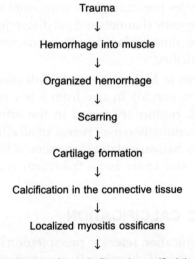

Trauma
↓
Hemorrhage into muscle
↓
Organized hemorrhage
↓
Scarring
↓
Cartilage formation
↓
Calcification in the connective tissue
↓
Localized myositis ossificans
↓
Replacement of muscle fibers by ossified tissue

There is no sex predilection for its occurrence. Often the individual gives history of traumatic injury in the past. In the radiograph, myositis ossificans appears as a homogeneous opacity involving the affected muscle.

Various other soft tissue calcifications to be considered in the differential diagnosis of myositis ossificans are mineralized stylohyoid ligament, sialolith, phlebolith and bone tumors.

Progressive myositis ossificans occurs rarely, especially in the infants. It is often associated with other developmental disorders. The bone formation occurs usually in the tendons and the fasciae.

The bone deposition usually begins in the neck and then the upper back and the extremities are involved. Often the condition begins as painful soft tissue swelling of the muscle. Radiographic features are suggestive of bone deposition within the involved muscle. It should be differentiated from localized myositis ossificans.

CYSTICERCOSIS

In cysticercosis (a parasitic infection caused by *Taenia solium*), the larval parasites penetrate the mucosa and enter the blood vessels and lymphatic channels and get disseminated. The dead larval spaces become replaced with connective tissue which may become calcified.

Usually there is history of gastrointestinal symptoms. Palpable masses, varying in size from a few millimeters to 1 cm in the neck region are noted in the affected patients. Radiographic examination may reveal small elliptical or ovoid calcified masses. Salivary gland stone should be differentiated from cysticercosis. There is no treatment required for this clinical entity.

DYSTROPHIC CALCIFICATION

Dystrophic calcification refers to precipitation of calcium salts in the primary sites of chronic inflammation and dead tissue, usually because of the activity of phosphatase enzymes. In the oral regions, dystrophic calcification is associated with swelling and ulceration of the overlying skin. In the radiograph, dystrophic calcification appears as irregular calcified outlines.

25 Chapter

Radiographic Features of Diseases of the Maxillary Sinus

- *Introduction*
- *Inflammatory Changes*
    Mucosal thickening
    Sinusitis
    Fluid level
    Empyema
    Polyps
- *Cystic Conditions*
    Mucous retention cyst
    Serous retention cyst
    Mucocele
- *Traumatic Conditions*
- *Tumors*

We pity you your sightless years,
And celebrate out learned day:
But Doris and the man in black,
With ancient wisdom, steal away.

– Ben Ray Redman

INTRODUCTION

The maxillary sinus begins to develop as an invagination of the epithelium of the lateral wall of the nasal fossa at about 3 months *in utero*. The size of the sinus is very small at birth and gradually increases in size until adulthood. The other paranasal sinuses are the frontal, the ethmoid and the sphenoid sinuses. The maxillary sinus is the largest and is located in the maxilla. The air-filled cavity is lined by pseudostratified columnar epithelium. The maxillary sinus is pyramidal in shape, the medial wall is formed by the lateral wall of the nasal cavity, the roof is formed by the floor of the orbit, and the floor is formed by the alveolar process of the maxilla. The maxillary sinus communicates with the nasal cavity through an ostium which is located near the top of the maxillary sinus, in some cases there may be an accessory opening posterior and inferior to the main opening (Fig. 25-1).

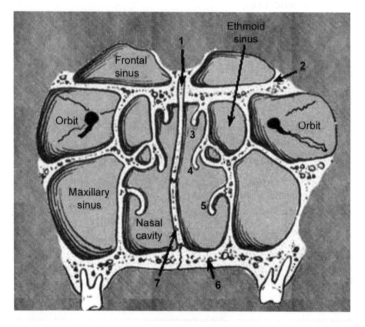

Fig. 25-1: Diagrammatic representation of maxillary sinus

Waters' view is the best radiograph in the evaluation of any pathology involving the maxillary sinus. Other radiographs that may be helpful in visualizing the sinus are periapical, occlusal, lateral skull and Caldwell projections.

Radiographic features of the diseases of the maxillary sinus can be broadly classified under the following headings.

I. Inflammatory changes
    i. Mucosal thickening
    ii. Sinusitis
    iii. Fluid level
    iv. Empyema
    v. Polyps.
II. Cystic conditions
    i. Intrinsic cysts
    ii. Extrinsic cysts
    iii. Mucocele.
III. Traumatic conditions
IV. Tumors
    i. Benign
    ii. Malignant.

INFLAMMATORY CHANGES

Inflammatory changes in the maxillary sinus may originate from dental or periodontal causes and due to nondental or nonperiodontal causes. The nondental or nonperiodontal causes for inflammatory changes are infections, allergies, chemical irritation, foreign bodies (e.g. displaced root tips) and traumatic injuries.

Various inflammatory changes involving the maxillary sinus are described below.

Mucosal Thickening

The thickness of the mucosal lining in a normal sinus is about 1 mm and is not visible in the radiograph. The thickness increases about 10–15 times due to infection or allergic conditions. A thickened mucosal lining may be visualized as an opaque band.

Sinusitis

Maxillary sinusitis is the inflammation of the maxillary sinus. It occurs usually as a sequel or complication of common cold and upper respiratory infections. In some cases maxillary sinusitis can occur as local extension of dental or periodontal infections.

Acute maxillary sinusitis is usually a complication of common cold. Patient reports nasal discharge, nasal congestion, pain and pain or heaviness while bending down. There can also be tenderness, elevation of temperature, and referred pain to the premolars and the molars.

Chronic maxillary sinusitis occurs as a sequel of acute infection.

Various radiographic changes observed are mucosal thickening, air-fluid level, and opacification of the maxillary sinus.

Fluid Level

Due to the fluid level, the translucency of the sinus will be lost at certain level in a horizontal direction. The main causes for fluid level within the sinus are pus caused by infection and blood due to trauma. Fluid level can be demonstrated by taking an additional radiograph by tilting the patient's head. If it is used to fluid level, even when the head is titled, it assumes a horizontal level.

Empyema

An empyema is a cavity filled with pus. This usually results from the blockage of the ostium. Empyema is usually associated with localized erosion of the bony wall.

Polyps

A thickened mucosa due to chronic inflammation may undergo polypoid hypertrophy, which is radiographically evident as a dome-shaped radiopacity. Polyps can cause alteration of the bone structure (either displacement or destruction), if the lesions are long standing.

CYSTIC CONDITIONS

Various cysts involving the maxillary sinus may be dental in origin (extrinsic cysts) or nondental in origin (intrinsic cysts).

The extrinsic cyst projects into the maxillary sinus. The extrinsic cysts are mainly the odontogenic cysts (periapical, dentigerous, keratocysts or primordial cysts). The intrinsic cysts are mucous retention cyst, serous retention cyst and mucocele.

Mucous Retention Cyst

Mucous retention cyst or cyst of McGregor is one which occurs as a sequel of hyperplastic mucosal lining of the sinus. Radiographically it appears as a ball-like radiopacity in the antrum without any cortical outline.

Serous Retention Cyst

The second type of intrinsic cyst is serous retention cyst. This cyst does not have an epithelial lining and consists of loculated and collected fluid in the mucoperiosteum. This cyst is inflammatory in origin. Radiographically these cysts are less radiopaque when compared to the mucous retention cysts.

Mucocele

Mucocele is a gradually expanding collection of fluid within the antrum, caused by the blockage of the ostium. There is usually expansion and thinning of the sinus wall and destruction and compression of the adjacent structures. Mucocele more predominantly occurs in the frontal and the ethmoid sinuses.

TRAUMATIC CONDITIONS

Maxillary fractures can involve the nose and the paranasal sinuses. Fracture of the floor of the maxillary sinus can occur during dental extractions. Radiographic evidences for traumatic injuries are fracture lines of the bony wall, displacement of fractured fragments and opacification due to the blood or the orbital contents. Oroantral communication is usually a complication associated with extraction of the maxillary posterior teeth. In the periapical radiograph it may be apparent as loss of cortical plate separating roots of the teeth and the antrum.

TUMORS

Benign and malignant tumors can involve the maxillary sinus such as fibrous dysplasia, ameloblastoma, central cemento-ossifying fibroma, Paget's disease, osteoma, epithelial papilloma and squamous cell carcinoma. As most of the tumors are discussed elsewhere, only the relevant tumors will be discussed here.

Epithelial papilloma is a tumor of the respiratory epithelium and occurs in the nasal cavity and the paranasal sinuses. Clinical symptoms are nasal obstruction, discharge, pain and epistaxis. Radiographically it may appear as a polypoid mass which is relatively radiopaque.

Osteoma of the maxillary sinus is an asymptomatic entity. Osteoma is usually seen in the frontal or the ethmoid sinuses. Osteoma can cause nasal obstruction and destruction of the bony wall. Expansile lesions can cause swelling. Radiographically it appears as a lobulated or rounded radiopaque mass.

Ameloblastoma, if it involves the maxillary sinus, appears as an expansion of the sinus and filled with soft tissue mass. Radiographically it may appear radiolucent with destruction of the bony elements.

Squamous cell carcinoma is a common neoplasm involving the maxillary sinus. Usually the affected individuals are over 40 years of age. The symptoms are nasal obstruction, discharge, bleeding and pain. Involvement of the orbit can cause epiphora (watering of the eyes) and proptosis (protrusion of the eyeball). The expanding growth may also be noticeable over the face or intraorally on the palate as swellings. There can also be hyperesthesia, anesthesia, trismus and obstruction of the eustachian tube causing stuffy ear.

Radiographic features are irregular radiolucencies and destruction of adjacent bony wall.

26 Chapter

Radiographic Features of Temporomandibular Joint Disorders

- *Introduction*
- *Developmental Disorders*
- *Enlargement of Coronoid Process*
- *Ankylosis*
- *Degenerative Joint Disease*
- *Rheumatoid Arthritis*
- *TMJ Osteoma*
- *Neoplasms*

Peace! Would you not rather die
  Reeling,—with all the cannons at your ear?
    So, at least, would I,
  And I may not be here
  To-night, tomorrow morning or next year.
  Still I will let you keep your life a little while,
    See dear?
  I have made you smile.

— Charlotte Mew

INTRODUCTION

Evaluation of the temporomandibular joint (TMJ) radiographically is extremely difficult. In Chapter 11 various TMJ views useful in the visualization of TMJ have been discussed. In this chapter various pathologic conditions involving the TMJ are discussed.

DEVELOPMENTAL DISORDERS

Various developmental disorders affecting the TMJ are condylar aplasia, hypoplasia, hypertrophy and hyperplasia.

Aplasia refers to the absence of the condyle. This is a very rare developmental anomaly.

Hypoplasia refers to smaller than normal size of the condyle. Clinically it is often associated with facial asymmetry. Various factors responsible for condylar hypoplasia are:
- Birth injury
- Radiation therapy at an early age
- Trauma
- Local infections
- Rheumatoid arthritis
- Hemifacial atrophy
- Scleroderma
- Postsurgical defect.

Radiographically condylar hypoplasia can be visualized as smaller than normal size of the condyle and malformation of the condyle.

Hypertrophy refers to increase in size of a part due to increase in size of the cells. It can be either idiopathic or associated with hemifacial hypertrophy.

Hyperplasia refers to increase in size of a part due to increase in the number of cells. Worth has divided condylar hyperplasia into three types. In type I, remodeling of the condyle results in condylar hyperplasia. In type II, there is no remodeling and the head of the condyle is replaced by a globular mass. In type III, the condylar enlargement may be due to an inflammatory process.

Hypertrophy and hyperplasia, when unilateral, cause restricted mouth opening, deviation of the mandible and facial asymmetry. Radiographically, condylar hyperplasia and hypertrophy are readily apparent as increased bulk of the head and the neck portions of the condyle.

Jonck has classified facial asymmetry into four types (Fig. 26-1).

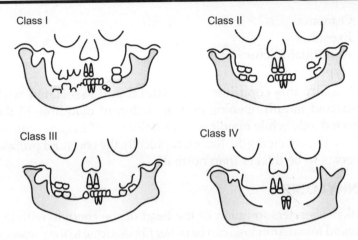

Fig. 26-1: Jonck's classification of facial asymmetry

According to this classification, class I and II are developmental in origin. The description of Jonck's classification is given below:

Class I   There are condylar enlargements, no midline deviation, and no loss of posterior occlusion.

Class II   Condyle and ramus are normal, there is midline deviation, there is elongated mandibular body and posterior occlusion is present.

Class III   In class III, the changes are acquired. The condyle is enlarged with spur formation, there is midline deviation and there is loss of posterior occlusion.

Class IV   In class IV, the condylar enlargement is due to neoplastic process. There may or may not be enlargement of the ramus and body and posterior occlusion.

ENLARGEMENT OF CORONOID PROCESS

Enlargement of the coronoid process is very rare compared to the condylar enlargement. Coronoid process may become enlarged due to:

• Osteochondroma

- Osteoma
- Exostosis
- Abnormal fracture healing
- Hyperplasia.

Usually this condition is unilateral and associated with restricted mouth opening and deviation of mandible to the affected side while opening. A prominence of zygoma can be felt on the affected side. Radiographically the coronoid process appears to be thicker than normal.

ANKYLOSIS

Ankylosis refers to union of the head of the condyle with the glenoid fossa. Ankylosis can be either fibrous (due to the presence of fibrous tissue) or bony (due to the presence of osseous structure). The causes responsible for ankylosis are the following:
- Birth injury
- Trauma
- Infection
- Rheumatoid arthritis
- Osteoma
- Neoplasms
- Prolonged intermaxillary fixation after fracture of mandible
- Surgical procedures involving the TMJ.

Bony ankylosis is radiographically discernible as lack of normal joint space and osseous mass at the TMJ region.

DEGENERATIVE JOINT DISEASE

Degenerative joint disease is also called as osteoarthritis, hypertrophic arthritis or arthritis deformans. It usually involves individuals over 50 years of age. In younger individuals it can occur due to chronic microtrauma as in the case of parafunctional habits such as bruxism and clenching and myofascial pain dysfunction syndrome (MPDS). The clinical symptoms usually reported by the patients are the following:
- Limitation of the mouth opening especially following long periods of inactivity
- Unilateral pain over the TMJ

- Clicking sound during condylar movement
- Tenderness
- Hypomobility
- Ear pain and headache
- Deviation of the mandible while opening the mouth.

Various radiographic features suggestive of degenerative joint disease are given below:
- Narrowing of the joint space
- Irregular joint space
- Facet formation on the condylar head
- Subchondral sclerosis
- Erosion of the condyle
- Cyst-like areas in the medial or the lateral aspect of the condyle (Ely's cysts)
- Osteophyte or spur formation.

RHEUMATOID ARTHRITIS

Unlike the degenerative joint disease, rheumatoid arthritis is an inflammatory joint disease and affects both the joints. Apart from the TMJ, many other joints are also affected. The clinical and radiographic features are essentially similar to degenerative joint disease. However, in rheumatoid arthritis, there is osteolysis of the condylar head. Juvenile rheumatoid arthritis (Still's disease) is associated with facial asymmetry.

TMJ OSTEOMA

TMJ osteoma is bony growth seen over the head and the neck of the condyle. It is usually associated with facial asymmetry and interferes with TMJ function.

NEOPLASMS

The main neoplasms that can involve the condyle are chondroma, osteochondroma and chondrosarcoma. Radiographic changes are similar to osteoma or hyperplasia and appear as enlargement of the head of the condyle. Other lesions involving the ramus and the condylar regions are benign chondroblastoma and odontogenic myxoma.

Infection Control in Dental Radiography

Behold,
  The time is now! Call in, O call
  The pasturing kisses gone astray
  For scattered sweets; gather them all
To shelter from the cold.
  Throng them together, close and gay,
And let me be the fold!

— **Alice Meynell**

INTRODUCTION

Infection control protocols are employed in dental radiography to reduce the potential for transmission of infectious diseases between patients as well as to those who handle the x-ray and related equipments as well as accessories. The possible modes of transmission of infection in dental practice are:
- From a patient to the dental professional
- From the dental professional to a patient
- From a patient to another patient.

Transmission of infection from one individual to another individual is due to the transfer of pathogenic microorganisms.

The dental professional and the patients are exposed to a variety of pathogens that are present in the oral or respiratory secretions as well as in the blood. These pathogens are:
- Cold and flu viruses and bacteria
- Cytomegalovirus (CMV)
- Hepatitis B virus (HBV)
- Herpes simplex, types I and II (HSV-I and HSV-II)
- Human immunodeficiency virus (HIV)
- *Mycobacterium tuberculosis*
- Fusospirochetes.

The transmission of infection may be due to the following reasons:
  (a) Direct contact with the pathogens in saliva, blood, respiratory secretions or lesions
  (b) Direct contact with airborne microorganisms in spatter or aerosols of oral and respiratory fluids
  (c) Indirect contact with objects or instruments contaminated with microorganisms.

The primary requisites for causing infections are:
- A susceptible host or a host with decreased immune status
- A virulent pathogen with sufficient degree of infectivity and numbers to cause infection
- Appropriate portal of entry for the pathogen to cause infection.

There are certain guidelines put forward by the Centres for Disease Control and Prevention (CDC) for effective infection control. These guidelines are given below.
- Vaccination of dental professionals especially against hepatitis B
- Thorough hand washing and care of hands from cuts
- Proper use and care of sharp instruments and needles
- Sterilization and disinfection of instruments
- Cleaning and disinfection of the dental unit and environmental surfaces
- Disinfection of the dental laboratory
- Use and care of handpieces and intraoral devices attached to air and water lines of dental units

- Single use of disposable instruments
- Proper handling of biopsy specimens
- Proper use of extracted teeth in dental educational settings
- Proper disposal of waste materials
- Implementation of recommendations.

The objectives of infection control can be achieved by the following means as proposed by Occupational Safety and Health Administration (OSHA):

1. Use of protective attire and barrier techniques
2. Handwashing and care of hands
3. Sterilization and disinfection of instruments
4. Cleaning and disinfection of dental unit and environmental surfaces.

PROTECTIVE ATTIRE AND BARRIER TECHNIQUES

This objective can be achieved by using protective clothing such as gowns, lab coat or uniform. Latex or vinyl gloves must be used during operative procedures. Surgical Masks and eyeglasses should be used to prevent spatter and aerosolized sprays of blood and saliva from causing infection, especially while using ultrasonic scalers and airotor.

HANDWASHING AND CARE OF HANDS

Proper care must be taken while handling sharp instruments to prevent pricks and cuts. Hands should be thoroughly washed before and after touching objects or surfaces contaminated by the blood or the saliva. Infected material should be prevented from coming in contact with cuts or wounds.

STERILIZATION AND DISINFECTION OF INSTRUMENTS

Based on the risk of transmitting infection, instruments have been classified into:

a. Critical instruments
b. Semicritical instruments
c. Noncritical instruments.

The critical instruments are extraction forceps, scalpels, scalers, surgical burs, etc. Dental radiography does not employ any critical instruments. The semicritical instruments are x-ray film-holders, mirrors, amalgam condensers, burs, etc. The noncritical instruments are position-indicating devices (PID) of the dental x-ray tube head, exposure button, x-ray control panel and lead apron.

Various sterilization methods are used such as autoclave (steam under pressure), dry heat, chemical vapor, and use of chemical disinfectants to sterilize nonautoclavable instruments.

The surfaces that have to be disinfected in dental radiography are:

X-ray Machine
Tube head, cone, control panel and exposure button should be covered or disinfected.

Dental Chair
The headrest, headrest adjustment and chair adjustment controls must be covered or disinfected.

Work Area
The area where x-ray films are placed during exposure must be covered or disinfected.

Lead Apron
The lead apron should be wiped with a disinfectant between patients.

The dental radiographer should wash the hands thoroughly between patients. He should also wear gloves, masks, and eyeglasses.

The exposed films contaminated with saliva must be properly handled. The films should be placed in a disposable container after drying the saliva.

The contaminated items must be disposed off in puncture-proof bags or containers.

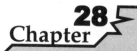

Chapter 28

Radiographic
Differential Diagnosis

- *Radiolucencies with Definite Borders*
- *Anatomic Radiolucencies*
- *Radiolucencies other than the Anatomic Radiolucencies*
- *Multilocular Radiolucencies*
- *Radiolucencies with Ill-Defined Borders*
- *Generalized Rarefactions*
- *Pericoronal Radiolucencies*
- *Localized Radiopacities*
- *Periapical Radiopacities*
- *Generalized Radiopacities*

CUT if any will, with Sleep's dull knife,
Each day to half its length, my friend,—
The years that Time takes off my life.
He'll take from the other end!

– Edna St. Vincent Millay

RADIOLUCENCIES WITH DEFINITE BORDERS
(FIG. 28-1)

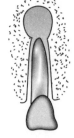

Fig. 28-1: Radiolucency with definite borders

ANATOMIC RADIOLUCENCIES

In the Maxilla

- Incisive foramen
- Superior foramina of nasopalatine canal
- Maxillary sinus
- Nasopalatine duct.

In the Mandible

- Lingual foramen
- Mental foramen
- Submandibular gland fossa
- Mandibular canal
- Mandibular foramen.

Common to both the Maxilla and the Mandible

- Bone marrow spaces and alterations in the trabecular pattern
- Tooth crypts in the early stages.

RADIOLUCENCIES OTHER THAN THE ANATOMIC RADIOLUCENCIES

- Extraction sockets
- Focal osteoporotic bone marrow defect
- Surgical defect
- Developmental lingual mandibular salivary gland depression (Stafne's cyst)
- Primordial cyst
- Lateral periodontal cyst
- Incisive canal cyst
- Globulomaxillary cyst
- Median mandibular cyst
- Residual cyst
- Traumatic bone cyst (solitary bone cyst).

Note: In the illustrations of this chapter, radiopacity is shown as black and radiolucency is shown as white for the ease of diagrammatic representation and better perception.

MULTILOCULAR RADIOLUCENCIES (FIG. 28-2)

- Odontogenic keratocyst
- Ameloblastoma
- Central giant cell granuloma
- Cherubism
- Odontogenic myxoma
- Aneurysmal bone cyst
- Central hemangioma of bone.

RADIOLUCENCIES WITH ILL-DEFINED BORDERS (FIG. 28-3)

- Osteomyelitis
- Osteoradionecrosis
- Primary intra-alveolar squamous cell carcinoma
- Central mucoepidermoid carcinoma of the jaws
- Metastatic carcinoma (from the breast, lungs, kidney, thyroid, prostate, colon and stomach)
- Langerhans cell disease (idiopathic histiocytosis)
- Multiple myeloma.

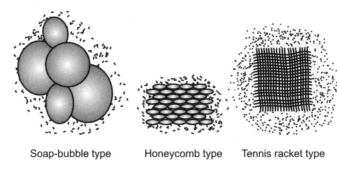

Soap-bubble type   Honeycomb type   Tennis racket type

Fig. 28-2: Multilocular radiolucencies

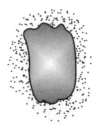

Fig. 28-3: Radiolucency with ill-defined borders

GENERALIZED RAREFACTIONS

- Hyperparathyroidism jaw lesions
  - Primary
  - Secondary
  - Tertiary.
- Osteoporosis
- Sickle cell anemia
- Thalassemia (Cooley's anemia)
- Massive osteolysis (phantom bone disease).

PERICORONAL RADIOLUCENCIES

With Radiopaque Flecks (Fig. 28-4A)

- Ameloblastic fibro-odontoma
- Adenomatoid odontogenic tumor
- Calcifying epithelial odontogenic tumor (Pindborg's tumor)
- Calcifying odontogenic cyst.

Without Radiopaque Flecks (Fig. 28-4B)

- Normal follicular space
- Osteitis with pericoronitis
- Dentigerous cyst
- Ameloblastic fibroma.

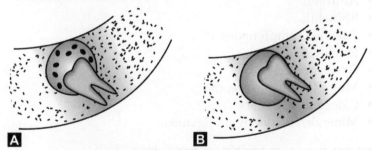

Figs 28-4A and B: Pericoronal radiolucency with (A) and without (B) radiopaque flecks

LOCALIZED RADIOPACITIES (FIG. 28-5)

Associated with the Jaws

- Exostosis
- Enostosis

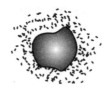

Fig. 28-5: Localized radiopacity

- Torus mandibularis
- Torus palatinus
- Idiopathic osteosclerosis
- Condensing osteitis
- Osteoma
- Chondrosarcoma
- Osteogenic sarcoma
- Foreign bodies
- Retained roots
- Odontoma (compound and complex)
- Ameloblastic odontoma
- Garré's osteomyelitis.

Not Associated with the Jaws
- Sialolith
- Antrolith
- Rhinolith
- Calcified lymph nodes
- Phlebolith
- Cysticercosis
- Multiple miliary osteoma
- Calcified acne scars
- Mineralized stylohyoid ligament.

PERIAPICAL RADIOPACITIES (FIG. 28-6)

- Idiopathic osteosclerosis
- Condensing osteitis
- Hypercementosis
- Periapical cemental dysplasia
- Benign cementoblastoma (true cementoma)

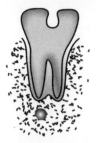

Fig. 28-6: Periapical radiopacity

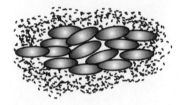

Fig. 28-7: Generalized radiopacity

- Benign osteoblastoma
- Central cementifying fibroma.

GENERALIZED RADIOPACITIES (FIG. 28-7)

- Florid osseous dysplasia
- Fibrous dysplasia
- Osteopetrosis (marble bone disease; or Albers-Schönberg disease)
- Paget's disease (osteitis deformans)
- Generalized cortical hyperostosis.

Further Reading

1. Oral Radiology Principles and Interpretation, Third Edition Paul W Goaz, Stuwart C. White. The CV Mosby Company 1995.
2. Differential Diagnosis of Oral Lesions, Third Edition, by Norman K Wood and Paul W Goaz. The CV Mosby Company 1985.
3. Radiographic Imaging. Fourth Edition, by Noreen Chesney and Muriel O Chesney. Blackwell Scientific Publications, the United Kingdom, 1965.
4. Panoramic Radiology, Second Edition, by Olaf E Langland, Robert P Langlais, W Doss McDavid and Angelo M DelBalso. Lea and Febiger, Philadelphia, 1989.
5. Stafne's Oral Radiographic Diagnosis, Fifth Edition, Edited by Joseph A Gibilisco. WB Saunders Company, 1985.
6. Radiology for Dental Auxiliaries, Sixth Edition, by Herbert R Fromer. The CV Mosby Company.

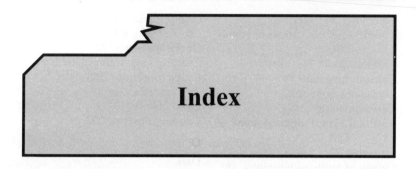

Index